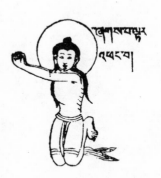

The Tibetan

Book of Yoga

Geshe Michael Roach

WITH THE DIAMOND
MOUNTAIN TEACHERS

Andrea McCullough
Winston McCullough
Christie McNally
Ani Pelma
Elizabeth Prather
Brian Smith
John Stilwell
David K. Stumpf
Susan Stumpf
Kevin Thornton
Miriam Thornton
Elly van der Pas
Douglas Veenhof
Rebecca Vinacour

Kimberley Anderson-Veenhof
Giselle Ansselin
Mercedes Bahleda
John Brady
Deborah Bye
Nancy Carin
James Connor
Ian Davies
Anthony Deague
Gail Deutsch
Michael O'Reilly Dunn
Rani Sheilagh Dunn (yogarani)
Alistair Holmes
Konchok Kyizom
Salim Lee
Anne Lindsey

doubleday
new york london
toronto sydney auckland

Ancient Buddhist

Teachings on the

Philosophy and

Practice of Yoga

The

Tibetan

Book of

Yoga

PUBLISHED BY DOUBLEDAY
a division of Random House, Inc.

DOUBLEDAY and the portrayal of an anchor with a dolphin
are registered trademarks of Random House, Inc.

BOOK DESIGN BY JENNIFER ANN DADDIO

Library of Congress Cataloging-in-Publication Data
Roach, Michael, 1952–
    The Tibetan book of yoga : ancient Buddhist teachings on
the philosophy and practice of yoga / by Geshe Michael
Roach.
      p. cm.
    1. Yoga (Tantric Buddhism)   2. Spiritual life—Buddhism.
I. Title: Ancient Buddhist teachings on the philosophy and
practice of yoga.   II. Title.

   BQ8938.R63 2004
   294.3'4436—dc21

                      2003053203

ISBN 0-385-50837-9

PRINTED IN THE UNITED STATES OF AMERICA

February 2004

First Edition

10 9 8 7 6 5 4 3 2 1

Contents

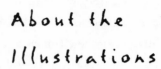

About the
Illustrations

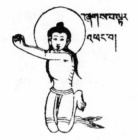

Throughout this book you will find a number of
traditional illustrations of yoga exercises and ancient masters
of the yoga tradition of the Dalai Lamas. Drawings like the one
above come from an extremely rare woodblock print that was
probably carved in Mongolia and is now held at the Oriental
Library of the Russian Academy of Sciences, St. Petersburg.

The carvings of important teachers of the tradition, with Tibetan captions below them, were completed at the Potala Palace of the Dalai Lamas before the fall of Tibet. The one illustration of the channels of the inner body is adapted from a series of yoga exercises in wall paintings discovered at the Lukhang meditation chambers of His Holiness the Sixth Dalai Lama (1683–1706). And, finally, the more boisterous drawings of yoga poses, without captions, come from the ancient Himalayan kingdom of Sikkim; they accompany a collection of yoga texts written in the 1700s.

Tibetan Heart Yoga in Photographs

The photographs in this book were prepared during a three-year deep retreat, undertaken by members of the author group in the Arizona desert. They show the major steps as you go through the half-hour practice. Be sure to also read the description of each exercise, for more hints and details.

The Tibetan
Book of Yoga

The Roots of Tibetan Heart Yoga

The ancient art of yoga came to Tibet from its birthplace in India over a thousand years ago. It quickly became very popular, and wonderful systems for its practice sprang up like mushrooms all over the country. The yoga practice you will learn here, which is called Tibetan Heart Yoga, belongs to the Gelukpa tradition of the Dalai Lamas of Tibet.

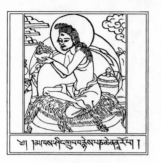

Master Naropa

Tibetan Heart Yoga works on your heart in two ways: It makes your physical heart and body healthy and strong, and it opens your heart to love others. And of course really the first always comes from the second.

The instructions for the physical exercises and inner practice of Heart Yoga entered Tibet in two different lineages. The exercises—or what we in the modern world think of as "yoga"—were first taught to Tibetans by the Indian master Naropa (1016–1110). They form part of an ancient tradition known as the Six Practices, and the Tibetans nicknamed them the "Machine of the Body."

The instructions for opening our hearts to others are called *tong-len*, which means "Giving and Taking." This practice involves special ways of breathing and thinking of others, throughout the day, and especially as you do your yoga exercises. The lineage for Giving and Taking goes back over two thousand years to the Buddha himself. It was passed on quietly from teacher to student without being written down and was brought to Tibet by the great Indian sage Atisha (982–1052). The practice was first put into book form by a Tibetan, Geshe Chekawa, about a hundred years later, and our presentation here is from his work.

Both the physical exercises and the special breathing techniques merged together by the time of Jey Tsong Khapa (1357–1419), who describes the yoga poses you find here in a secret text called *The Book of Three Beliefs*. The three beliefs, by the way, are belief in the beauty of the way; belief in the one who teaches it to you; and belief in yourself, that you will succeed in your practice.

Jey Tsong Khapa was the teacher of His Holiness the First Dalai Lama (1391–1474), and from here Tibetan Heart Yoga continues up to His Holiness the current Dalai Lama, whose cheerful wisdom and compassion certainly embody its goals. Those of us who have written this book received the instructions on Heart Yoga over many years from great Tibetan lamas, especially Khen Rinpoche Geshe Lobsang Tharchin and Sermey Jetsun Geshe Thupten Rinchen. They in turn received them chiefly from Kyabje Trijang Rinpoche, the teacher of His Holiness the Dalai Lama. Thus it is an authentic yoga you will learn here, and we hope that the blessings of this long line of masters will touch you, even if we ourselves as teachers are but mere babes by comparison.

The daily half-hour program for Tibetan Heart Yoga presented in this book is both similar to and very different from other kinds of yoga being taught today. On one hand we have selected exercises that you are probably already familiar with if you have ever tried yoga; you will feel at home here whether you are just starting out or whether you are already attending classes in the Ashtanga, Iyengar, Shivananda, Jivamukti, Bikram, or another common yoga tradition. We ourselves enjoy and practice these well-known programs too; this book was in fact written during a deep three-year retreat in the Arizona desert, and

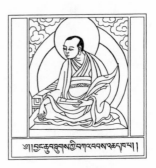

Geshe Chekawa

throughout this time we received training in these five systems by kind and dedicated teachers who traveled far to come and instruct us, often at their own expense.

Each of the standard yoga poses you find here is accompanied by an additional pose that will be new for you; these are from the book by the teacher of the First Dalai Lama. These exercises deepen and strengthen the effect of their sister poses. But the most important difference between this yoga tradition and the others is in how you breathe and what you think about as you do your exercises. The Heart Yoga of Tibet works from both the inside and the outside, to bring you lasting strength and calmness. So next let's take a look at how this happens.

> Come to understand
> That great core
> within you,
> Like the very axis
> Around which
> the stars turn.
>
> —The *Yoga Sutra* of Master
> Patanjali (3rd Century)

How Heart Yoga Works

Most of us are interested in yoga because we hope that it will give us more energy, better health, a trim and more flexible body, and of course peace of mind. Most of us too are more likely to really put our heart into a daily program like this if, at the very beginning, someone can give us a clear idea of how it works. To understand how helpful Heart Yoga can be, you need to understand what we call the Five Levels.

Think of your body like an onion. On the outside are all the parts we can see: arms, legs, tummy, and such. When we do yoga, this outer layer is what we think about the most. Where am I supposed to put my foot? Where does my arm go? Am I finally looking better?

And then there's a second layer right below the first. This level is made of all the things that give our outer body energy to be healthy and strong. One example of course is what we eat, but the ancient books of the East say that other things sustain our physical body as well—things like hope, and sleep, and even quiet times when we can sit down and think about something without being interrupted.

The most important source of food, raw energy for our bodies, is not what you might expect; it is our very breath. We can go for days without eating, or even drinking, but a good gulp of breath is something we need every couple of seconds. Our bodies contain billions of cells, and each one is fed consistent meals of fresh oxygen through the wondrous network of our lungs and bloodstream. If our breathing is deep and steady, it nourishes us automatically; we glow with health. And so of course all systems of yoga emphasize staying aware of our breath as we move through the exercises.

But now when you peel off this second layer, the breath, you come to a third level: one that makes the breath itself move. And this is the inner winds. Think of pictures you've seen of how the nerves spread throughout our body, branching off from the spinal cord like limbs of a tree, reaching out to the ends of our hands and feet.

Our nervous system really counts as part of the first level: the outside body. Now imagine a ghostlike network of tiny pipes and channels made of stuff so fine that you could no more touch it than you could grab a ray of sunlight peeking in through your window. This is what we call the inner channels—they lie inside the whole framework of nerves and blood vessels and even bones within our body. In fact, you could say that the very patterns of

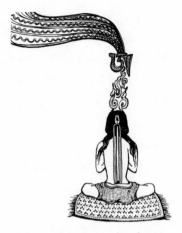

The inner channels, from the meditation chamber of the Sixth Dalai Lama

our nervous system and veins and skeleton all grow within us, in the first place, by following the outline of the lightray channels that are already there, even in the womb.

The whole shape of our body then, inside and out, is simply a reflection of the shape of these subtle inner channels. Have you ever gone outside in the sun in the morning after an ice storm and seen the branches and twigs of every tree in your yard coated in beautiful glistening ice? The shape that the layer of ice on each twig takes all depends on the shape of the twig beneath it: If the twig has a bump, then the ice forms a bump over it.

Every bump and indent on the outside and the inside of our bodies then is a reflection of a twist or turn of the invisible inner channels. The bones of our lower back, for example, form in the shape they do because there's a very similar, lumpy intersection of the inner channels right there in the same space.

You can probably already guess where all of this is heading. If these same inner channels lying within your lower back get knotted up somehow, then the very bones of your lower back get jammed up too. And that's exactly what causes a sore back. So if you really want to fix the pain in your back, you need to fix the problem at the level of the inner channels: at the third level.

Although people might not talk a lot about these inner channels in a typical yoga class nowadays, the whole purpose of yoga exercises in olden times was to reach down to this third level and straighten out problems with the inner channels. And because the first and second levels rest upon this third level, your breathing and your health straighten out as soon as the inner channels do.

All of this so far is working on yourself from the outside, with the yoga exercises. Now we get to the exciting part, which is the special secret of Tibetan Heart Yoga: working from the inside.

Working from the Inside

Blood flows within the network of our veins, and tiny electrical impulses pass through the branches of our nervous system. What is it that moves within the inner channels?

It's the inner winds. They're called "winds" because, like the wind that propels a sailboat, they are invisible to the eye but very powerful nonetheless. They also have a strong connection to another kind of "wind," and that's our own breath as it blows in and out of us.

Think of the inner winds and your breath like a pair of strings on a guitar. If you tune two strings to exactly the same note, then you can pluck one and the other one vibrates all on its own. Your breath follows your inner winds like that. If the inner winds are flowing calm and easy, then the breath too flows the same.

But what makes the inner winds flow? For the answer to that, we need to peel off another layer of the onion and go down to the fourth level.

The fourth level is, quite simply, your own thoughts. Thoughts and the inner winds are always connected; they run in tandem, the thoughts riding on the winds like a rider on a horse. This connection between our thoughts and the winds within the channels is the amazing border where our body meets our mind. And this too is where Tibetan Heart Yoga does its work.

You can trace this connection yourself simply by thinking about the last time you got really excited or upset. When we have a strong emotion like this, then our thoughts stop flowing smoothly; they literally get jumbled up. And because the thoughts ride on the horse of the inner winds, then the winds also start to struggle inside the channels. It's as if a rider suddenly starts kicking and digging spurs into a horse's side. The horse takes off in any direction it wants.

And because of that connection between the inner winds and our breath, like two guitar strings, then the breath goes out of control too. We start breathing faster and faster, in fits and starts.

Suddenly the cells in our body aren't getting their meals on time. Keep this up long enough, and it causes an ulcer or a heart attack, or maybe just wrinkles: The body is telling you that you haven't treated it right.

And so really a moment of strong negative emotion at the fourth level, the thoughts, disturbs the inner winds that are linked to our thoughts. This problem at the third level reverberates on the second one: our breath. And that creates trouble at level number one, which is the health of our bodies. Trouble at level four works its way up to level one.

If you think about it, this whole process provides us a wonderful opportunity as well: We can take advantage of the interconnection among all these levels to fix things. And that's really what most types of yoga aim at. You stretch and pull at the physical body, which makes your breathing deep and regular. This settles down the inner winds, which automatically calms the thoughts that ride on them. It's like grabbing the reins of a runaway horse and bringing it to a gentle stop. The rider atop the horse comes to a stop too, simply because he's on top. This is exactly why a good yoga session leaves us feeling calm and refreshed.

But what if we go at it the other way around: What if we work from the inside? Suppose we could figure out the very most beautiful thoughts of all, the ones that flow in the most perfect way of all. Then we could sit down quietly and—well— just think them, very much on purpose.

Since the inner winds are tied to these same thoughts, then

the winds would start to flow calm and free within the inner channels. This would trigger the same change on the next level up: We'd start to breathe slow and free too. The cells all get their meals right on time, plenty to eat. That makes the body bright and slender and strong. And we did it all just with our thoughts. That's the key to Tibetan Heart Yoga.

> What? Did you think
> That heaven and hell
> Were built by a
> construction
> company?

—Gautama Buddha (500 B.C.)

World-Seeds

We started out talking about five different levels. What happened to the fifth one?

It's all very well and good to tell people that if they think calmer thoughts they'll feel better physically; we knew that already. The problem is that we usually don't have any choice about it. Problems come up in our lives, with situations or the people around us, and make it difficult to be calm or peaceful all the time.

One solution we spoke about already: When you feel tired, upset, or unhappy, you can always get on your yoga mat and go through the exercises. You sweat, and the effect works its way down to the inner winds and your thoughts. You feel better for a good while afterward, and that in turn is good for your body's health.

The real question though is all about the fifth level. If the inner winds drive our breath, and our thoughts drive the inner winds, well then what is it that drives the thoughts themselves? Why is it that certain things can make us upset in the first place? And where did all these things come from anyway? To understand this, we need to understand what the ancient books call "world-seeds."

Three people go to their first yoga class. An hour later one of them walks out with a strained neck. The second didn't find the class very interesting, and never comes back. The third person goes home feeling light and full of energy, delighted to find a fun, new way to stay healthy and trim. All three of them took the same class; all three did the same exercises. So why the difference?

If you think about it, the yoga class was only one thing. But three different people experienced it as three different things. The masters of old say this comes from the different world-seeds in each person's mind.

What's a world-seed? It's a little seed in our mind that ripens when we look at something, and colors how we see it—like putting on a pair of red-tinted sunglasses and looking at a piece of white paper. Then the paper is pink.

World-seeds decide how everything in our whole world looks to us, good or bad. If a good world-seed is ripening in your mind when your boss walks in the door, you see her come up to you and offer you a raise. If a bad world-seed is ripening, you see her yelling at you. She's the same boss, she's only one boss. How you see her depends on which pair of sunglasses the world-seeds in your own mind have put on your nose.

Where do these world-seeds come from? How do they get planted in our minds? The answer is the same from women and men of wisdom throughout history, in every part of the world: You get what you give; what goes around comes around. Call it karma, or simply reaping what you sow. The seeds that determine how we see our world are planted in our minds by how we treat other people.

Think of your mind as a sophisticated video camera. When you say or even think something unkind to someone else, your own mind records the event. Depending on how strong your emotions were at that time, a seed of certain power is planted in your mind. A week later, or maybe a month, whatever, the boss walks in the door. The world-seed wakes up and gives you a terrible pair of sunglasses and you see . . . the boss yelling at you.

If you've been kind, instead of nasty, to someone else, then a different world-seed ripens and you see yourself getting a raise from the very same boss. You get the picture (if you have the seeds to).

Let's go back to the three people who took the same yoga class, with three different results. According to this idea of getting back what you give to others, the person who walked out with a sore neck did so because at the very bottom level— at the fifth level—a seed woke up in his own mind and made

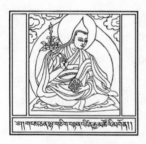

Portrait of the
current Dalai Lama
as a young man

him experience the class that way. And he planted the seed by, say, ignoring a friend at work the week before who needed an aspirin for a bad headache.

The second person, the one who didn't feel too much one way or the other about the yoga class, didn't have any strong good or bad seeds waking up. And the third person, who may have gone to visit a sick friend the week before, comes out of the class feeling like a million dollars, because that world-seed has ripened for her.

These world-seeds are very powerful things. They bubble up from the fifth level all the way to the first and decide how our body responds to yoga. And they go further still, shaping our very life and world as we go.

So in a way then the future ahead of us is like a blackboard with nothing written on it. You can almost think of it like the nothing that's at the very middle of the onion, after you peel off the very last layer. Whether yoga works for each of us—what we're going to see on the blackboard—depends on us.

Now this whole idea of world-seeds, that you get back exactly what you give, is as old as history. But somehow it gets a little hard to believe on a personal level. You don't have to worry much about that now, just keep it in mind as we go; let's see if it really works. It's a big part of how Tibetan Heart Yoga "does its thing" to give you a trim, healthy body and a cheerful mind throughout the day, just like that Dalai Lama with his big irrepressible smile.

To sum up what we've said so far, we're looking for a yoga

program that works on all five levels at once, because that would be five times more powerful than just a simple yoga class. We want a yoga that can stretch and loosen the right places in our body; make our breath calm and full; get our inner winds flowing smoothly; fill us with good and kind thoughts; and help us plant seeds in our mind for a beautiful future world. And that's exactly what half an hour of Tibetan Heart Yoga does for you every day. So let's get on with the first exercise.

EXERCISE • 1 •

The

Diamond

in the

Rose

Here we begin the first of the ten exercises of Tibetan Heart Yoga. Each time we do a new exercise, there will be instructions first on how to do it. Then we'll explain how the exercise actually works on your body and mind, bringing strength and calmness, from the first level all the way down to the fifth.

How to Do the Exercise

- Time: 2 minutes.
- Sit comfortably at the front of your yoga mat.
- Join your palms at your heart with the thumbs side by side, in between your hands. Press into your chest.
- Close your eyes lightly, and focus your mind quietly at the spot between your eyebrows.
- At your heart, picture a red rose. Lying in the middle of the rose is a sparkling diamond.
- Now softly sing the words "Om mani padme hum" (pronounced *Om mani pay-may hoong*). Or, if you wish, use any other brief line that uplifts and inspires you. Keep your mind on the picture of the diamond in the rose until the time is up.

How the Exercise Works on You

The point of this first exercise is to warm and loosen the inner channels in the area of our heart. This quiet singing or chanting is not just a silly thing that some people go through at the start of a yoga class. It's as important to do before yoga as warming up is before you go jogging. Let's see why.

We've spoken about a network of channels, channels made of light, that provide the foundation for every part of our body. The most important of these channels runs up and down the very core of our body, like the great invisible axis that our dear planet Earth spins around. Whenever the inner winds flow freely within this channel, we feel bright and happy.

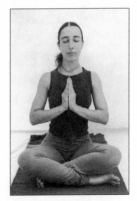

Meditation

Alongside this central channel, to the left and the right of it, run two other channels. They are a little smaller, and at certain points they cross over and around the main channel like vines twisting around a stick of wood. The winds that flow inside these channels are connected to our negative emotions: anger, desire, selfishness. Any time we think a negative or harmful thought, it stirs up the winds within these two side channels, again because our thoughts and the winds are like a rider upon a horse.

When the winds in the side channels are stirred up, these channels begin to expand, like long thin balloons as you blow air into them. The side channels then begin to choke the central channel, at the places where they twist around it. This in turn starts to block the free flow of wind in the main channel, like a garden hose with a kink in it. And because all our good thoughts are linked to the winds in the central channel, we begin to feel nervous or unhappy. Since trouble at one level touches all the other levels, our physical health is affected.

The most serious tie-up point of all lies in our central channel at the level of our heart. Here the two side channels twist around the main one most tightly, which is exactly why your chest might start to hurt after a few especially stressful days at work, or with your family. All the exercises of Heart Yoga are targeted at this blockage point at the heart, opening it up in order to free thoughts of happiness and nourish the body.

Singing or chanting has an especially powerful effect on loosening this tie-up of the channels at the heart. This is why it's so hard to sing when we're in a grumpy mood; we already have a knot in our hearts. It's also why so many of us enjoy singing in the shower: The central channel actually runs closer to our back than to the front of our bodies, and a warm spray of water can loosen this area. This relaxes the crossover point at our heart and makes us feel like singing.

You've probably guessed by now that the whole reason the heart has been connected to feelings of love and kindness over the centuries all goes back to loosening up this particular knot around our central channel. I give my heart to you; open your heart; may you have all that your heart desires. The exercises of Tibetan Heart Yoga are based on something we've known all along about our hearts.

So singing is good for our heart; now, what shall we sing? The small chant here is very, very old and has been the favorite of all the Dalai Lamas. Imagine all the good and kind thoughts that have been thought so far today, inside the heads of every single person in the world. Now imagine that we could put all these thoughts in one place and build a person out of them, like a snowman made of handfuls of snow. It would be some

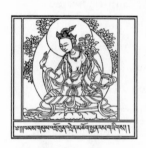

Loving Eyes

kind of exquisite being of pure perfect light, like an angel in the old paintings.

The Tibetans thought of this beautiful creature as an angel they called Chenresik, which means the Angel Who Looks upon Us with Eyes of Love, or simply Loving Eyes. They believed that each of the Dalai Lamas was in reality this angel. Be that as it may, the small chant we use here has always been connected with the angel Loving Eyes and thus with the Dalai Lamas. It has a very special effect upon opening the tangle at our hearts.

The song of Loving Eyes is written in Sanskrit, the ancient language of India. The sounds of Sanskrit lie at the bottom of about half the languages of the world, including English. The Tibetans believed that this is because the words we use for things all came originally from the deep and subtle sounds of the winds running within our own bodies. Sanskrit is based upon these windsongs. So when we sing in Sanskrit, it helps release the tie-ups of our inner channels. The sound of *om*, for example, opens us up to be more kind to others in our actions, words, and thoughts.

Lots of us might feel more comfortable doing the chant in our own language, and that works well too. In English the words come out as "I sing the diamond in the rose." The original words mean "Om, the jewel in the lotus," but in Heart Yoga we use the diamond and the rose, for a very special reason.

The flower here in our hearts is meant to be one that is lovely and fragrant, and also one that thrives under difficult circumstances. In India this is the lotus, a pink-orange bloom with a subtle but striking perfume. A lotus always grows in the dirtiest, most polluted part of a pond, rising gracefully out of the filth, untouched by it. The flower represents our love for others, the love in our

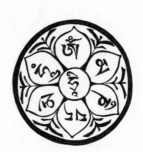

The Song of
Loving Eyes

heart, which grows calmly and unaffected even during the most stressful and difficult moments of our day.

When you picture the bloom within you, it's important to use a flower that you grew up with, since it moves your subconscious thoughts and winds more strongly. For most of us then the red rose is best, growing as it does with almost no water, even in the desert, even in a busy modern life.

We picture the diamond within the rose because, on the day that the knot in your heart opens completely, you will see a clear crystal light reaching out from there in love, to every living thing in the entire universe. And behind this love is the ultimate truth of all things, itself as pure and indomitable as a diamond.

As the Dalai Lama often says during his talks around the world, it is also very appropriate during this first exercise simply to chant the name of any special being, past or present, who has meant a lot to you during your life. It could be Moses, Jesus, or Muhammad; or a dear teacher from school; even the name of your mother or father, wife or husband. Anyone who inspires in you the feeling of heart-kindness.

Don't be shy; sing out clear and long. It's a little corny, but it's very important if you want the yoga to make you trim and strong. When the two minutes are up (you might want to set a timer), then go on to the second exercise.

A person whose
mind is wandering
Has already put
their head
Between the jaws
of the terrible
Lion of unhappiness.

—Master Shantideva
(8th Century)

EXERCISE ·2·

The

Perfect

Ten

In the second exercise we watch our breath, to bring the mind within and allow us to focus on the yoga exercises to come. These instructions are taken from a book by the First Dalai Lama called *A Lamp for the Path to Freedom*. They in turn come from the *Treasure House of Wisdom*, written by the Indian master Vasu Bandhu over sixteen centuries ago.

How to Do the Exercise

- Time: 2 minutes.
- Sit comfortably at the front of your yoga mat.
- Place your hands on your knees, palms up.
- Softly touch the thumb of each hand to the first finger. Relax the other fingers.
- Straighten your back, make sure your shoulders are level. Loosen any tightness in your forehead and the corners of your mouth. Keep your chin up straight—not too high or too low.
- Gaze downward and then softly shut your eyes.
- Take a breath, and then let the air out through your nose, long and slow. From here on, breathe only through your nose.
- Now inhale gently. This exhale followed by an inhale counts as one breath. We call it one cycle of exhale/inhale.
- Concentrate on your breaths up to ten. Start over if you find yourself thinking about anything else.
- When you reach ten, or the time is up, go on to exercise three.

How the Exercise Works on You

Our breath is tied to our inner winds, and our inner winds are tied to our thoughts. This means that when we have kind or peaceful thoughts, then our breathing too becomes calm and regular. It also means that if we consciously breathe in a very regular way, then our thoughts will become quieter. And that is something very important if we want the Tibetan Heart Yoga exercises to make us stronger and more healthy.

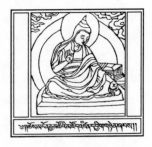

Master Vasu Bandhu

The physical poses of yoga are meant to stretch and straighten the inner channels, which allows the winds to run more smoothly. This effect at level three rebounds back up to our body at level one and makes it trim and fit. But if we do the yoga exercises while we are worrying about a problem at home or at work, then that jumbles up the inner winds, again because of the connection between the thoughts and the winds. And then whatever good result we might have gotten from working on the outside, with the exercises, is canceled by the turmoil of the winds on the inside. Yoga done with a wandering mind is a lot like not doing yoga at all.

The ancient masters of yoga recognized this and made Perfect Ten a requirement before going on to the physical exercises. The name "Perfect Ten" comes from the fact that you have to be able to count ten silent breaths perfectly—which means without thinking about anything else at all.

Once you try this, you'll discover that it's not at all as easy as it sounds. Imagine your mind sitting on the end of your nose like a guard at a bank vault. Feel the breath coming and going at the very opening of your nostrils. As you get better at this exercise, you can also start to listen for the very tiny sound of the breath passing through the fine hairs inside your nose, like wind through the trees. Later on you'll be breathing so gently that even this soft sound fades away.

If you catch your mind thinking about anything else during the ten breaths, then start counting over again, at breath number one. If you're very honest with yourself, you'll probably find that it's difficult to reach even three or four before your mind goes off to something else. This is an undeniable sign of just how distracted the modern mind is. If we are unable to still the mind even when we really want to, then our inner winds must be in a constant state of rush and confusion.

It's very important to realize that, according to the ancient books, this turmoil of our thoughts and inner winds is responsible not only for ill health, but also for the process of aging itself. So if you know how to work with your inner winds properly, you can actually turn the clock back.

A few details about how to do the exercise: It's good if you can cross your legs, because this makes it easier to keep your back straight

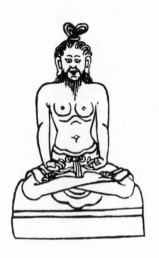

than if you have your legs stuck out in front of you. A straight back is absolutely essential for the winds to flow properly in your central channel. This is exactly why you can think more brightly and clearly when you're sitting up straight in a chair: As the winds flow, so flow the thoughts. It's also why so many of the exercises here are aimed at making your back more strong and flexible, especially in the crucial area of the spine right behind your heart.

As your yoga practice progresses, you can begin to sit in the half-lotus posture, with your right foot up on your left thigh. Later on you can even try the full lotus or the *siddha asana*: the sage's posture. These you should learn from a qualified instructor, someone who can check and see if your knees have been loosened up enough first by the yoga exercises.

To help keep the back straight, Tibetan masters often recommend using a small cushion under the back part of your seat, so that the area at the base of your spine is up higher than your thighs.

If you find that closing your eyes all the way makes you drowsy, then try opening them just a bit—but continue to gaze downward, and avoid focusing on anything in front of you.

Perhaps the most important detail of the Perfect Ten concerns how we count our breaths. Normally when someone tells us to start counting breaths we take a deep breath in, as if we were about to swim some distance underwater. Then when we let the breath out again, we think of that as the first breath, and we go on counting like that.

But it's a unique feature of Heart Yoga that we always count our breaths beginning from the out-breath first. This way of breathing will continue throughout all of the yoga exercises here; it's very important to think of a "breath" not as breathing in and then out, but rather as breathing out and then in.

For one thing, this way of breathing makes it a lot easier to calm your breath down—try it and see. If your breath has speeded up or fallen out of rhythm because you're nervous or upset about something, it's almost impossible to quiet it down very quickly by consciously trying to force yourself to breathe in more calmly. But if you focus on slowing down the out-breath, if you just try to let the air out in a long, slow, complete flow until your lungs are empty, then your breathing settles down right away.

Think about how your breath feels when you release a good sigh. And here we're not talking about the explosive kind of sigh that bursts out when you're very tired, or exasperated with somebody. We mean that slow gentle sigh that comes up out of your chest and the bottom of your throat when you're feeling very contented and relaxed; the kind that just sort of slides out all on its own when you're lying on a couch listening to your favorite music, or when someone gives you a hug. You can also think of how children breathe out while they sleep.

This is how we want each breath in Tibetan Heart Yoga to start—with this same soft sigh as the breath flows out. If you get used to thinking of a breath this way, as one cycle of an exhale followed by an inhale, you'll find that it makes you calmer throughout the entire day. So begin to work on it here, during the Perfect Ten.

There's another reason why we breathe with out-breaths first, and then in-breaths. The first breath we ever took, as we came out of our mother's womb, was an in-breath. And the last breath that people take, lying on their deathbed, is an out-breath. Yoga, as it was meant to be by the ancient masters of India and Tibet, is a protest against this normal way of things. We don't need to get old the way we do, they say. We were meant for life and not for death. Let the last breath out come first and then let us breathe in—let us live. Let the inner winds flow free into the central channel, and sing there always.

> Giving and taking
>
> Ride on the wind
>
> Freeing every
>
> living being
>
> From the sea
>
> of pain.

—The First Panchen Lama
(1567–1662)

EXERCISE ·3·

Taking Away the Darkness

Here we begin what is certainly the most important exercise of Heart Yoga. Of all the yoga exercises we could do, this one has the most profound effect at the deepest level: the fifth level, which is made of the seeds that create our very world and body.

How to Do the Exercise

- Time: 3 minutes.
- Continue to sit comfortably at the front of your yoga mat, after finishing the Perfect Ten breaths.
- Bring your mind into the spot between your eyebrows. This time, move your focus up from this spot half an inch toward the top of your head. And then go about an inch *into* your head. This is a perfect place to gather your concentration.
- Now bring your thoughts down to your heart again. Go very deep into the heart, to a place an inch or two in front of your backbone.
- See there the diamond in the rose. It has always been there. Smell the fragrance of the flower, and gaze upon the sparkling clearness of the crystal.
- Next think of someone you love—friend or family—whom you know is going through some kind of physical or emotional pain right now. Try to picture clearly the room in which the person is sitting.
- Now imagine that you have gone to sit just in front of this person. You are invisible; they can't see you, but you can see them.
- Now pretend that all the pain this person has, in body or in mind, has gathered into a little pool of darkness at her or his heart. It looks like a small cloud of black ink, about the size of a coin.
- Pause here for a few moments and think about how the pain feels to your loved one. Think of the different worries that

must be going through her or his mind right now. Be specific; get to the details. Your mind will want to wander off—bring it right back to their problem.

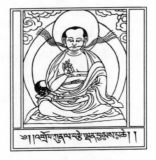

Giving and Taking

- Think about how wonderful it would be if you could take away the pain. But what if the only way to do that were to have this same pain yourself? Decide that you would be willing to do even this; it is the kind of decision that brings true meaning and happiness to our whole life together on this Earth.

- Decide then without any doubt or hesitation that you will take the person's pain away and take it upon yourself. We do this by taking several deep in-breaths. Each time we breathe in, the little cloud of darkness moves a little farther, carried by this gentle wind. It slowly moves up our loved one's throat and then out of her or his nose in a black stream, like cigarette smoke.

- This stream of darkness collects in a little cloud again, just in front of your own nose. Pause and take a few quiet breaths, to get ready for one last in-breath. This is the one that will actually bring all the pain into you. Be brave and decide again that it would be better if you hurt, than them.

- Take one last moment to look at the diamond in the rose. The diamond is sparkling, radiant with light and power. It can destroy anything that touches it.

- It's absolutely crucial at this point that you think about how the power of the diamond is going to destroy all of the darkness, in the very same instant that you breathe in the little cloud. This is because our very willingness to take on someone else's pain destroys all of that pain forever, for both them and ourselves. Never think for a moment that any of that darkness will be left inside of you.

- With a single breath in now, see the darkness come into your nose like a stream; it collects in a tiny ink-black cloud just in front of the diamond; and then it touches the diamond—all in a single in-breath.

- The moment that the edge of the cloud touches the edge of the shining diamond, there is a sudden explosion of golden light throughout the inside of your body. It's as if a very powerful photo flash has gone off within you, at your heart.

- After the flash, all you can see is the diamond, lying lovely within the rose, glistening as it always does. You see a tiny wisp of white smoke vanish into the air, and all the pain is gone. It is very important to see that all of the pain is gone. Nobody will be hurt by this pain now, ever again.

- Sit for a few moments more, quietly, until the time is up. Again you are sitting in front of that same friend or family member, and you are still invisible. Just rest here for a moment, silent, and enjoy the look on the person's face. Suddenly all the pain and trouble your loved one has been having is completely gone. They don't know why, but they don't really care. How good it feels now! Enjoy your loved one's happiness, and be proud of yourself, that you had the courage to take their pain away.

How the Exercise Works on You

We all want to be happy. It is the reason why every single one of the billions of people around our world put their feet on the floor and get up out of bed in the morning.

And in our pursuit of happiness during the whole day that follows, we can all end up doing some pretty selfish things, even things that might hurt the other people around us. But this is not who we really are. This is not what we really want to do, and we know it. And it happens that we often get back in our bed at night less happy than when we started out in the morning, searching for happiness.

To put it very simply, the one thing that makes every one of us really happy is making other people happy. We just forget this sometimes, in the rush of life. And that's why we do the ancient practice of Giving and Taking every time we do Tibetan Heart Yoga. We do something to make someone else happy; and there's nothing in the world that can make us happier too.

Actually, the taking part of Giving and Taking always comes first. We do the giving part later, because it's more fun to get a gift from someone after you're feeling better than when you're still quite ill.

Taking away other people's pain is the very heart of Tibetan Heart Yoga. To understand why, we have to go back to those five levels.

Twisting ourselves up like a

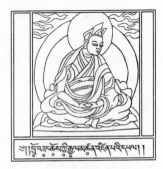

The First
Panchen Lama

pretzel in a yoga class sometimes only goes as deep as the first level, especially if we haven't been taught the various poses in the correct way—in the way of the ancient teachers. That is, you may feel better physically for a while, but it doesn't last.

The traditional yoga exercises, done the right way, are designed to reach down to the second and third levels: They help bring the inner winds back to a smooth flow, which makes our breath flow calmly and smoothly too. This sweet breathing then resonates back toward the inner winds, making them even more smooth. Health at this deep level inside us bubbles up to the first level and, with regular yoga practice, makes us feel lighter and younger physically.

Even this effect though doesn't necessarily reach the fourth or the fifth level: our thoughts, and the world-seeds within our own mind. And this means that no really permanent improvement in our health will happen. If yoga isn't done at these two deepest levels, then we just get old while we do yoga to feel younger. And then after a certain number of classes, over a certain number of years—no matter how disciplined we've been with our yoga practice—we get old. To be frank, we grow too old even to do any more yoga; and this happens *while* we do our yoga. But it doesn't have to be that way.

We all know, deep inside, that what really makes us happy is to make other people happy. The best kind of thought that a human brain can think in a whole day is the inspiration to do something that makes someone else happy. So suppose we spend a few minutes even just imagining how nice it would be if we could take away some of the pain that someone else is going through. It's just so good and right that our very thoughts begin to sing within the inner channels.

This has an immediate effect on the levels above it; the inner winds connected to our thoughts begin to sing too. That in turn triggers a song in the breath itself, and this brings a steady flow of delicious air to the cells of our body. And then the yoga that we do will really work on us. We won't be the one that leaves yoga class with a sore neck; we'll be the one who goes home feeling like a million dollars.

But the most exciting part of Giving and Taking is what it does to the level below our thoughts: to the world-seeds at the fifth level. Even just two or three minutes of being good to someone else—even just a few minutes of *wishing* we could be good to someone else—plants a huge basket of very pure, very powerful seeds within our own mind.

And remember that, when these seeds sprout, they determine how we see everything in the world around us—even how we see ourselves. If we've planted bad seeds in the past, by ignoring what others need, then we'll see the boss walk in the door and yell at us. But if we've planted good seeds—say by doing the ancient practice of Giving and Taking while we do our yoga—then we see the boss walk in and give us a raise. Or maybe we just see ourselves getting a whole lot healthier from the yoga. And then, you see, we can make this little fantasy of Giving and Taking come true after all; we can show others how to do what we ourselves have done.

Don't ask yourself,
"If I give this away
To someone else,
what will I
have for me?"
Instead ask yourself,
"What is the
use of having
something,
If I can't give it
away to
someone else?"

—Master Shantideva
(8th Century)

EXERCISE · 4 ·

Giving

with

the Sun

Now we are truly prepared to do the physical yoga exercises; now they will really work on us, reaching all the way down to the fifth and deepest level. We begin with that old yoga favorite called "Bowing to the Sun" (*Surya Namaskara*), but we do it in a very new and special way, from the lineage of the Dalai Lamas.

How to Do the Exercise

- Time: 5 minutes.
- Stand at the front of your mat, with your feet together.
- Inhale, then say quietly, "I give you the gift of giving." Join your palms at your chest, and close your eyes. Inhale again.
- Stand still now for five cycles of exhale and inhale. Breathe very slowly and fully, and only through your nose. The rose with the diamond inside it is still there at your heart, fragrant and sparkling. Each time you breathe out, the air you release carries the lovely scent of the rose. This scent surrounds you now.
- Think again of that special person in your life—the one whose pain you took away during the last exercise. Go again and sit in front of the person. Now that we have removed all their worries, we want to fill her or him instead with good and happy thoughts. The first thought is simply a very great willingness to give things to other people. We are going to send our friend the gift of giving itself. Once they receive it, they will suddenly feel the joy of giving. They will suddenly want to give all kinds of things to others—whether it be material things like money, or protection from fear and trouble, or love itself, or even the understanding of how to work at all five levels and find lasting health.
- Each time you breathe out now, imagine that the warm fragrant scent of the rose leaves your nostrils. It comes softly into the other person's nose; they breathe it in, and the air travels down to their own heart. See now another red rose

and diamond inside of them. Suddenly the person feels the joy of wanting to give, give to others, all they need.

- With this joy, the diamond at your loved one's heart glistens, like a pure pool of light-blue water caught in the moonlight. Rays of sky-blue, water-pure light sparkle from both diamonds—yours and theirs—and form a bridge of light between your hearts. Sometimes then your diamond even sinks into theirs, as one, in silence.

- After the fifth in-breath this way, we are ready to begin the physical yoga exercises. From here on every single breath will be accounted for—there will be no extra breaths, and we will be doing something very specific on each out-breath and each in-breath. At first you will need to set aside a few additional moments and breaths to check what comes next in the book. Within a week or two it will all be automatic. Remember that it's very important now for you to think of "a breath" as one out-breath followed by one in-breath, and not the other way around. Keep your mind on this throughout the exercises.

- *Out-breath:* Now join your palms at your heart with the thumbs inside, hooked together. Press your hands into your chest and take the first out-breath.

- *In-breath:* Keeping the hands together, straighten your arms out in front of you, and then drop them together toward the floor. Now reach with straight arms all the way up to the sky and a little behind you, arching back gently. Bend at your heart, not at your neck or lower back. Gaze straight upward, not back at your hands. (See top photo, page 44.)

- Hold this position for five cycles of exhale/inhale. This is the Tibetan pose called "Sky Diamond" (*Namka Dorje*).

- *Out-breath:* Now swing your arms back down in front of you as you fold your chest to your legs. Hold your ankles, or else hold your big toes with your first two fingers, keeping your legs and back straight. Then as you progress, try to place your hands on the floor beside your feet. Gaze toward your feet.

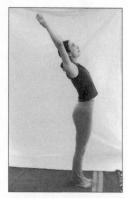

Bowing to the Sun,
Sky Diamond

- *In-breath:* Step straight back with your left foot about three feet. Keep the left leg straight, and bend your right leg at the knee.

- *Out-breath:* Step the right foot back next to the left one, and raise your hips up to the sky, keeping the legs straight. Press down into the floor with your hands and feet, and gaze toward your navel. (See bottom photo, opposite.)

- *In-breath:* Lower your hips and move your chest directly over your arms, making a straight plane with your body from head to feet—as if you were about to do a push-up.

- *Out-breath:* Bend your elbows, slowly lowering your body toward the floor. Keep your chin up and gaze straight ahead.

- *In-breath:* Push your body forward with your hands, rolling onto the tops of the feet. Then straighten your arms and arch back, gazing upward. Remember to bend at the area of the heart, and not so much at the neck and lower back.

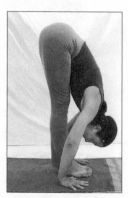

Bowing to the Sun,
folding down

- *Out-breath:* Push yourself back up again to the position where your hips are raised and your hands and feet are pressing into the floor. Gaze toward your navel.

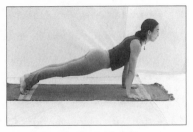

Bowing to the Sun, straight plane

- *In-breath:* Step your left foot up between your hands, keeping this leg bent and the right one straight, and turning your right foot out slightly. Join your palms together with the thumbs hooked inside, and raise your arms straight up. Gaze up toward your hands, arching slightly at the heart and not the neck.

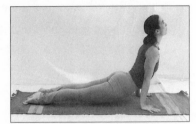

Bowing to the Sun, arching up

- *Out-breath:* Place your hands down again on the mat, on either side of your front foot. Then take that foot back next to the right foot, again making a straight plane with your body. Bend your elbows and lower your body toward the floor, gazing ahead with your chin up.

- *In-breath:* Push your body forward with your hands, and roll onto the tops of your feet. Then straighten your arms and arch back, gazing to the sky.

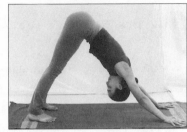

Bowing to the Sun, pressing down

- *Out-breath:* Push yourself

back to where your hips are raised and your hands and feet are pressing into the floor. Gaze toward your navel, and hold for five cycles of exhale/inhale.

- *Out-breath:* Step your left foot up between your hands in a lunging motion, gazing straight ahead.
- *In-breath:* Step your right foot up beside the left one, and straighten your legs and your back as if you were taking a bow. You are still gazing straight ahead.
- *Out-breath:* Bring your gaze down to your toes, grasp your ankles, and bring your chest toward your legs, keeping them straight.
- *In-breath:* Join your palms together with the thumbs hooked inside, bend your knees slightly, and reach with straight arms up to the sky again. Arch back gently at the heart, gazing straight up.
- *Out-breath:* Straighten up to a standing position, bringing your joined palms back to your heart, with the thumbs side by side between the hands.
- Repeat the entire sequence, but this time step with the right foot first.
- Repeat both sides one more time.

How the Exercise Works on You

With this exercise, and throughout the rest of the exercises to come, we begin the giving part of the traditional practice of Giving and Taking—the key to Heart Yoga in the tradition of the Dalai Lamas. This giving is done as we exhale our breath; we are combining perfect thoughts with our physical breathing, which is a little like touching a match to a bowl of gasoline. There is an immediate and powerful effect on both our health and our peace of mind. Let's see how this effect travels across the five levels.

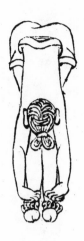

The reason that Bowing to the Sun is such a powerful yoga exercise is that it actually combines a number of traditional poses together, in a fun way, which gives us all the benefits of each one. Standing at our mat in the beginning—called "Mountain Pose" or "Steadfast Pose"—gives us a sense of balance and straightness. This feeling of a steady axis going through the center of our whole body is actually a tiny touch of the power of the central channel. The inner winds begin to stir there simply because of our good posture.

When we lift our arms up to the sky, tension in the neck and shoulders is released. This release is in fact due to a slight opening of two blockage points in the inner channels: one at the base of the neck and another near the backbone behind the heart. Because Heart Yoga stresses opening the heart, we pause here to take five slow breaths, out and then in.

It's very important to focus on bending backward at this area of the spine behind the heart; don't bend your neck back very far, and do try to keep your lower back almost straight. If you take the bend behind your heart and hold it there, you get a much more powerful effect on opening the constriction at the heart.

The forward bend at our waist that follows helps immensely to remove excess fat at the waistline. It's important to keep your head straight, and bend from your hips and not your lower back.

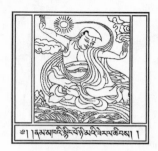

Riding the Sun

A qualified yoga teacher from almost any tradition can show you how this is done, and that's another beauty of Heart Yoga: You can "piggyback" this practice on top of whatever you're learning at your local yoga center.

The forward bend also helps release tie-ups of the inner channels near the spine just above your waist, and also down closer to your tailbone. This improves our digestion—gradually you'll feel a natural craving for healthful foods and less desire for unhealthful ones. You'll also just naturally feel like eating less than you used to, because your digestion is working at its optimum capacity. This in turn makes you more trim and strong: There is less of you to carry around all day, and less of the body's precious energy is spent on breaking down and digesting extra food—food that will never get used by the body anyway and just passes out.

The release of the channels here also affects your sexual life, giving you more energy in a clean, healthy way. This is because the improvement of the flow of the inner winds below our waist is reflected by a greater calmness and pureness in the thoughts. Then you can really channel all this sexual vitality into every part of your life; you become more creative and have tons more energy every day.

The push-up motion that comes next strengthens the chest and lower back; your arms will also begin to look more attractive, whether you're a woman (more slim and trim) or a man (a sculpted muscle look). This is followed by another back bend of the spine as you pull your head and chest up to the sky. Again, try to push your chest out and take the bend behind your heart, not in the lower back. One trick here is to consciously pull your shoulder blades toward each other in the back and also to be aware of the skin stretching in front, across your chest.

The upside-down V-shape that we make next, by sticking our bottom up in the air, acts as a counterpose to the backward bending of the back we've done. This stretches the back sides of the vertebrae, to even out the stretching of their front side—thus preventing soreness in the lower back. And of course this soreness occurs in the first place because of that tie-up of the inner channels at this same spot. The stretch helps relieve the knot.

The reach to the sky with spread legs and a bended knee, finally, increases strength in the legs, and makes them more shapely as well. The spread itself helps open up a knot in the channels at the area of the groin, again contributing to digestive and sexual energy.

Each time you reach to the sky in this exercise, be sure to hook your thumbs together inside your palms, and think of the gesture as the rose and the diamond in your heart. This constant reminder actually helps open the heart.

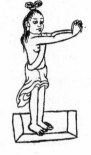

Now the entire exercise so far is really working on our blockage points from the outside; again, the real secret of Heart Yoga is what we do from the inside—which is infinitely more powerful. Throughout the exercise, with every exhale counting as the beginning of a breath, we try to keep our mind on giving something precious to the person we are trying to help—to the one whose pain we took away before.

This brings us to the idea of a checklist within our own mind—something like the checklist that pilots or astronauts go through before they take off, to make sure everything is working right. We've mentioned before that yoga doesn't work very well for us if, as we do it, we let our minds wander aimlessly through all the problems and plans of our daily life. This is because the inner winds get jumbled up if our thoughts do. Often a yoga teacher might tell us to watch our breath as it goes in and out during the entire yoga session. This, and gazing steadily at an outside spot like our fingertips or a smudge on the wall, can be very useful in "staking down" the mind, keeping it focused, as we do the exercise.

But frankly, it can get a little boring if you try to think only of your breath or a spot on the wall for the whole session. Inevitably your mind will start wandering off to something else. So take advantage of the situation, and let it wander to your mental checklist.

This checklist is a way to keep your yoga practice getting better and better all the time. It's a list of things you want to stay aware of during your yoga session; things that will help you improve and make the most of your precious time. The list can include some very important standard items that never change, and then some specific points that you're working on at the time.

The specifics list might include items like "Am I opening my shoulders the way my yoga teacher asked me to during that last class?" The standard list could go like this:

1) How is my breath? Am I concentrating on exhaling first and then inhaling?
2) Am I making the sighing sound as I breathe out, slow and long?
3) Is my face relaxed, smiling, and happy?
4) Am I gazing steadily at the proper spot and then moving my eyes smoothly to the next spot?
5) Am I stretching my body long and thinking that I'm straightening the inner channels?
6) But most important: Am I remembering to send my gift to that special person every time I breathe out?

Again, at first you won't be able to keep any one of these points in your mind for very long as you go through each yoga exercise. At the beginning, a lot of our effort is expended just trying to put a foot or a hand in the right place. In fact, the first few weeks of learning yoga are the hardest; a beginner is working much harder than someone with more experience. So you have every reason to be proud of yourself for your hard work, during the first few weeks especially.

Once you're moving along fairly well, then begin to go through this mental checklist constantly during a session. Your mind will still wander, especially if you're having a difficult week at work or something like that. But every time you catch yourself, bring your mind back calmly and with good humor to the checklist. Nobody's perfect; we know this even from the stories of great yoga masters from ancient India and Tibet. So don't let yourself get too serious.

The crucial item on every checklist is to see if you're still sending help to that special person as you breathe out. If you keep this up, then beyond any doubt your yoga practice will bring you everything you ever wished for, and a lot more.

During this particular exercise, Bowing to the Sun, we are sending out the gift of giving. We are giving someone else the strength to be generous, whether with money, or help, or love, or knowledge—knowledge of the kind that could change a person's life for the better, knowledge like an understanding of the five levels, and how to use them to become strong and calm.

You'll find over time that imagining you could send someone else generosity, just by breathing out, begins to have a deep effect on your own life. Every time we think of helping someone else become more generous and giving, we plant very powerful seeds within our own mind. As the seeds ripen, we ourselves become more giving people.

This then triggers a major change in the free flow of our thoughts and the inner winds they ride upon. That simply makes us more and more contented and joyful. And because of the connection between our inner winds and our breath, we begin to breathe more deeply and calmly throughout the day. This in turn makes our body strong—strong in such a way that you'll soon find that you almost never get sick anymore, and have plenty of energy all day to do the things you want. This makes us happier, and then the cycle between the five levels starts over again, going higher and higher. That's how Tibetan Heart Yoga makes all the difference, no matter what kind of yoga exercises you're learning.

EXERCISE •5•

Kindness
from
the West

The fifth exercise begins with the Western Stretch
(*Paschimottana Asana*), one of the most important yoga exercises
of all from ancient Indian books like *A Lamp for the Yoga of the
Sun and Moon* (14th century). "Western" here refers to the back,
because yoga is good to do facing east—the direction in which
we turn as we stand on Earth. And so it's a stretching out of the

back, and especially of the central channel running along the spine.

The accompanying Tibetan pose here is the Diamond Wheel (*Dorje Korlo*), which has the most pronounced effect of all on the spine behind the heart. The description for this and the following exercises in the tradition of the Dalai Lamas is from Jey Tsong Khapa (1357–1419), the teacher of the First Dalai Lama.

How to Do the Exercise

- Time: 4 minutes.
- After the last breath of the previous exercise, sit down on your mat as you exhale. If you need to, take another breath or two to get settled, stretching your legs out in front of you.
- Press your palms down on each side of you, to help you sit up straight.
- Inhale, then say quietly, "I send you kindness."
- Sit silently for five cycles of exhale/inhale, sending the breath and light.
- *Out-breath:* Begin the Western Stretch, by bending over and grasping your ankles. As you become more flexible, try to grasp your big toes with the first two fingers of each hand.
- *In-breath:* Arch back, opening the heart, as you pull back on your ankles or toes.
- *Out-breath:* Lower your chest toward your legs, leading with your heart.
- *In-breath:* Gaze softly at your big toes as you hold the pose.
- Remain here for five cycles of exhale/inhale.

- Release the pose as you exhale and sit up.
- On the next in-breath, cross your legs into a comfortable sitting position, and interlock your fingers behind your back, keeping your arms straight.
- *Out-breath:* Now begin the Diamond Wheel, turning your upper body to the left and at the same time bringing your clasped hands to the right. Turn your head and gaze over your left shoulder

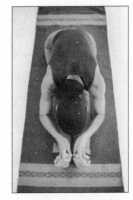

Western Stretch

  as far as possible, holding the pose for five cycles of exhale/inhale. Concentrate on turning the area of the back behind the heart, not the neck or lower back.
- *Out-breath:* Release the turn and come back to center. Take a breath.
- *Out-breath:* Turn your upper chest to the right, taking your clasped hands to the left. Turn your head and gaze over your right shoulder as far as possible, holding the pose for five cycles of exhale/inhale.
- *Out-breath:* Release the turn and come back to center.
- *In-breath:* Interlock your fingers directly over your head, keeping the arms straight and gazing ahead. Pull upward with your hands and lengthen your spine.
- *Out-breath:* Keeping your arms straight and your body lengthened, lean to your left side. Hold the pose for five

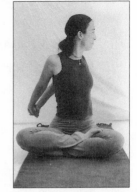

Diamond Wheel, turn

cycles of exhale/inhale. Be very sure to bend at your heart, not at your neck. Keep your lower back straight.

- Take a breath out, then inhale and raise up to center.
- *Out-breath:* Keeping your spine lengthened, lean now to the right side, holding the pose for five cycles of exhale/inhale.

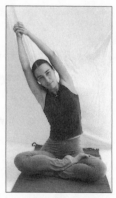

Diamond Wheel, lean

- Take another breath out, and then inhale and come back up to center.
- *Out-breath:* Interlock your fingers behind your back with your arms straight, and lower your heart toward the floor in front of you, keeping your back straight. At the same time, raise your arms up to the sky. Keep your forehead parallel to the floor so that your spine is as straight as possible from the top of the head to the tailbone. Hold the pose for five cycles of exhale/inhale.

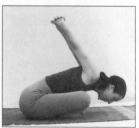

Diamond Wheel, fold

- Take a breath out and then inhale and sit up straight.
- *Out-breath:* Keeping your fingers inter- locked behind your back, pull your hands backward until the heart raises up and you arch back gently. Tilt your head back slightly and gaze to the sky, holding the pose for five cycles of exhale/inhale. As

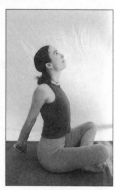

Diamond Wheel, arch

always, concentrate the bend at the heart, not the lower back or neck.

- Exhale and release the pose.

How the Exercise Works on You

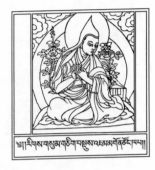

Jey Tsong Khapa, Teacher of the First Dalai Lama

The two poses in this exercise have a two-step physical effect. The front bend over our legs is one of the best ways to open up the knot in the inner channels within the lower back. Again, this knot is ultimately the reason why so many of us have trouble with our lower back in the first place. In a tiny form, the knot is present in the body even during the first few moments of life, just after the sperm of the father combines with the egg of the mother.

Thoughts at a subconscious level, connected to inner winds, are already jamming up then at the knot. The bones of our inner back gradually form around the knot, already one of the weakest and most vulnerable points in our body's framework. This exercise helps open the knot, which we need to do if we want to open the corresponding knot at our hearts.

This is because there is an affinity between the tie-up points in our body—much like the interconnection of the five levels themselves. Just as breathing more calmly triggers a better flow in our inner winds, a loosening of one of the major knots in the body triggers a loosening in the other knots. Working at the lower back does half the work at the heart.

The real work at the heart comes with clasping our hands

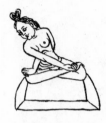

behind our back. This automatically opens the chest; again, try to push your shoulder blades together in back, to enhance the effect. As you turn to the side, consciously try to turn not only your neck and lower back, but also the area of the spine behind your heart.

This area is one of the most difficult to open, because the vertebrae in our spine behind the chest are different from the other vertebrae in our back. These particular vertebrae are attached to our ribs: They have to carry the whole weight of the cage that protects our heart and other vital organs of the chest. As a result, there is less mobility here in the back, and the channels can become almost stagnant.

Raising our clasped hands overhead and bending them to either side stretches this normally immobile area. Again, try to take the bend in the back behind the heart, and not very much at all in the lower back or neck. It's not a question of how far over to the side you can bend; that doesn't matter at all. The important thing is to feel the bend in the bones of the spine behind the heart.

After this we bend frontward over our legs again. Keep your concentration on stretching the whole back out as long as you can, and on pushing your chest out ahead as far as it will go. The goal of these forward bends is not to touch your head to the floor—if you push that way you'll probably just tighten the knot at the lower back instead of loosening it. Go down gradually, keep the back very straight, and keep your heart bursting out ahead.

At the beginning, your tummy will get in the way on the bends to the front. After a few weeks of this exercise, the inner channels get the message and begin to expel the extra body fat here. This makes you trimmer, lighter, and more comfortable all day long. That makes you happier, which affects the inner winds, and you set off another upward cycle in your life.

Bending backward at the end of the exercise, again stay aware of bending that stiff section of spine right behind the heart, and not so much at the lower back or neck. Remember throughout the exercise to go through your mental checklist. Does each breath begin with a full, steady exhale? Is my gaze fixed on a single point? Why did that lady at work yell at me today? Oops, back to the checklist. What am I giving to that special friend right now, with the fragrant breath of the rose, and the diamond light?

The gift during this exercise happens to be kindness, or—to put it more basically—simply not hurting other people. This all goes back to the fifth level, the level of the seeds that create our world. As the Dalai Lama often notes, every great religious teacher who ever lived has tried to convince the rest of us not to hurt one another. And our yoga practice doesn't have a hope of helping us if we don't really understand why.

Suppose we get upset at someone and say something that would hurt their feelings. Even during the few seconds that it takes to say the words, our ears are open and hearing ourselves speak: We hear ourselves hurt the other person, we see the reaction in their face.

All this action is recorded by that video camera of our own mind, which is turned on 24 hours a day. Each separate image of how the other person's face falls is recorded—dozens of pictures are snapped before we even finish the sentence. Each shot is stored in the mind and festers there, like a seed underground in springtime.

Sooner or later the seed ripens in our own thoughts and colors how we see all the people and things around us. We won't experience our neck as feeling light or flexible after yoga class; instead, we'll experience it as feeling sore. So if we really want yoga to *work* on us, we have to have what the Dalai Lama calls "enlightened self-interest" during all our interactions with other people. We can't do, or say, or even think anything that might hurt someone else, because everything is picked up by our own video recorder and gets played back to us later on.

Even a single
moment of anger
Destroys years
of kindness
to others.

—Master Shanti Deva
(8th Century)

EXERCISE • 6 •

The King of Patience

In ancient India, the first part of this sixth exercise was called the "King of Fishes Pose" (*Matsyendra Asana*). Matsyendra is the name of a great Indian master who lived over a thousand years ago; his teachings on yoga, and those of his disciple, Goraksha Natha, had a strong influence on the yoga lineage of the Dalai Lamas.

The second part of the exercise is perhaps one of the most distinctive poses of the Tibetan tradition, and is called "the Hook" (*Chakkyu*).

How to Do the Exercise

- Time: 4 minutes.
- Sit up straight, keeping your legs stretched out in front of you.
- Inhale, then say quietly, "I send you patience."
- Sit still for five cycles of exhale/inhale, sending the light and breath.
- *Out-breath:* Begin the King of Fishes Pose by bending your left knee and placing your left foot outside of your right knee. Then bend your right knee, keeping the outside of this leg on the floor and the right foot beside your left buttock.
- *In-breath:* Bring your right elbow to the outside of your left knee, then reach down and hold your left foot with your right hand.
- *Out-breath:* Turn and gaze over your left shoulder, reaching your left hand around your back and resting it as close as you can to your right thigh. Then hold the pose for five cycles of exhale/inhale. Concentrate on turning behind your heart, not with your neck or lower back.
- *Out-breath:* Release the turn, facing front and taking an in-breath.

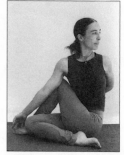

King of Fishes

- Repeat this sequence to the opposite side.
- Then release the turn and again extend your legs straight in front of you. Sit up with your back straight and exhale.
- *In-breath:* Now begin the Hook by interlocking your fingers in front of your heart, bending your elbows out to the sides.
- *Out-breath:* Thrust your clasped hands out straight in front of you in one quick motion. Hold there and take a breath in, lengthening your spine.
- *Out-breath:* Turn to the left, and take your arms to the left as far as you can without bending them. Turn your head and gaze toward your hands, holding the pose for three cycles of exhale/ inhale. Again concentrate the turn behind your heart.
- *Out-breath:* Now bend your left arm, placing the elbow against your left side, and pull your arms even farther to the left. Take your gaze over your shoulder as far as possible, holding this pose for three more cycles of exhale/inhale.
- *Out-breath:* Release the turn and face to the front. Then repeat this sequence to the right side.

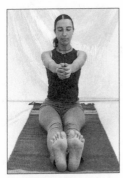

The Hook,
preparation

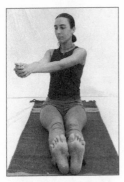

The Hook, straight
arm turn

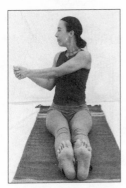

The Hook, bent
elbow turn

How the Exercise Works on You

The effect of this exercise again travels in two steps. The first part releases a special tie-up in the area of the hips, which once more invigorates your sexual and digestive energy. This particular combination of poses is interesting because the increased flow of inner wind frees physical air trapped in the stomach and intestines. So don't be surprised if you find yourself belching or passing gas as you go through the turns; it's a good sign.

The turning motion also tightens the abdominal muscles, flattening your stomach and removing excess fat at the waistline.

As you move into the Hook, the loosening effect moves up to the critical points of your upper back at the heart, as well as the neck and shoulders. At the base of the neck, near the spine, is another major knot. That's where stiff necks come from in the first place. When this tie-up is relaxed, it echoes back to the knot at our hearts—the main target for Tibetan Heart Yoga.

Stay aware of your gaze as you turn; keep it coming up in your mental checklist. Consciously forcing your eyes to look to the side, as far as you can, relieves tension and fatigue in them; you'll gradually find that this improves your eyesight during the whole rest of the day.

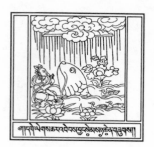

King of Fishes

Keep in mind too how your breathing, at level two, provides a bridge between the yoga exercises and your inner winds, so all these good things can happen. It's important to turn your upper body only as far as you can and still breathe comfortably; don't let the breath jam up as you hold the turn. Each time the breath comes back in, consciously try to pull up your spine: straighter and longer.

You can take advantage of this connection between the first three levels if you work for extended periods during the day at a desk, or in front of a computer. The tie-up point in the back of the hips tends to compress when we sit for a long time without standing or stretching. The inner winds start to back up, and you'll notice that your breath gets shallow and shaky. When you finally do stand up, your back is sore. This exercise helps loosen the blockage, restoring full breathing and flexibility of the hips.

Hips play an underrated role in the health of our whole body; as you do your yoga practice regularly they will start to open up, and then you'll find simple actions like walking or sitting a pleasure. The hip knot is opening, singing to the knot at the heart.

Down below the inner winds, our thoughts are flowing more freely too, first because they're tied to the freer flow of the winds. But sending the gift to that special person is working on these winds too, from the inside. This time we are sending the gift of patience. This is the power not to get angry at those specific moments during the day when something really pushes your buttons.

The teacher of the First Dalai Lama says there are two kinds of patience that you can send. One, of course, is patience with people whom you find it difficult to be around: Your boss at work could well be an example. But another kind of patience is simply not getting

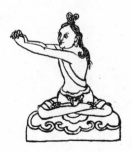

upset at events and situations: a headache, a traffic jam, or bad weather outside.

The trick is to catch yourself at the very early stages of anger, just as you begin to feel a little off-balance or annoyed. After this has grown into full-blown anger, which can happen in a minute or two, it's usually too late to control yourself. And a moment of anger can destroy all the good that months or years of kindness and friendship have built.

By the way, here's a little trick you can do sometime if you know you've got a particularly tough day, or even a week, ahead of you. Maybe you're supposed to go to a meeting later that morning at work with someone who often upsets you. The ancient books on Giving and Taking say that you can also send the fragrance of the rose and the light of the diamond— patience itself—ahead into the future to *yourself*.

The effect of doing this is quite amazing; try it sometime. Right in the middle of the meeting, just when the other person begins to get difficult, you'll suddenly find yourself receiving a big dose of patience: calmness and a smile. You may not even remember where it came from.

When I say that you

should work hard,

All I really mean is

that you should enjoy

Doing good things

for others.

—Master Shanti Deva

(8th Century)

EXERCISE · 7 ·

The Bow
& Arrow
of Joy

There is a logic by tradition to the order in
which we do the exercises; certain joints are better loosened up
after others, certain knots are easier to approach once others
have been breached. We are warm enough now to work directly
on the heart with a full backward bend of the spine, using the
well-known pose called "the Longbow" (*Dhanur Asana*).

This is complemented by a Tibetan pose named "the Arrow" (*Datar Sang*), which also provides a countermovement to the front. It brings us back to center and prevents any soreness after the session. The Arrow also incorporates an old Indian pose called "the Lion" (*Sinha Asana*), a secret weapon in removing tension and fatigue.

How to Do the Exercise

- Time: 3 minutes.
- Sit up straight, then say quietly, "I send you joy."
- Sit quietly for five cycles of exhale/inhale, sending the light and breath.
- *Out-breath:* Begin the Longbow by lowering yourself to the floor and turning over to lie down flat on your stomach. Then take a breath in.
- *Out-breath:* Bend your legs, then reach behind and grab your ankles.
- *In-breath:* Pull forward with the arms and backward with the legs, raising your chest and thighs off the floor. Then hold the pose for five cycles of exhale/inhale.
- *Out-breath:* Lower down to the floor and release the pose. Take a breath or two, then repeat.
- *In-breath*: Now begin the Arrow. Raise up to your knees, keeping them about two feet apart, but with your

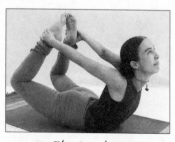

The Longbow

feet touching each other. Flex your feet so that your toes are flat on the floor, and balance on your knees and toes. Then sit down gently on your heels. Take a breath out and in if you need to, to get settled.

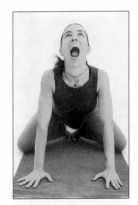

The Arrow, arch

- *Out-breath:* Place your hands on the floor between your knees, with your fingers pointing forward. Now arch your upper spine back, pushing your heart forward, and tilt your head up, gazing to the sky. Open your mouth and bring your jaw down, stretching the facial muscles. Hold this pose for five cycles of exhale/inhale, still through the nose.

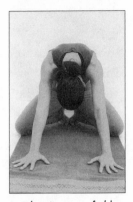

The Arrow, fold

- *Out-breath:* Now lower your head down and round your back, pushing into the floor with your hands to stretch your heart. Hold here for five cycles of exhale/inhale, but this time send each breath out sharply through your mouth, making a whisper sound of "ha."

- *Out-breath:* Sit up and release the pose.

How the Exercise Works on You

In our everyday lives, we rarely have any reason to arch our spine back, the way you would if you looked up to follow a plane passing straight overhead. And so age and the pressures of life gradually work the bones in our back over the other way, until we're stooped over and sunken in the chest. This closes the heart up like a clam. The seventh exercise of Heart Yoga turns this process back the other way.

Go very slow and easy as you persuade your back to open up backward. It took years to get that slight stoop into your spine, and it takes a while of gentle, steady practice to straighten things out again.

In the beginning, you might want to use some extra padding under your hips—a folded blanket is fine. Men especially might need to take an extra breath or two to rearrange matters under their shorts. Otherwise, the pressure you feel against the front of your lower abdomen is a good thing—it actually helps flatten your belly and stimulate glandular activity.

Again, focus on opening your chest and heart. Push your shoulders back, and take the bend behind your heart. Sometimes if feels more dramatic to force the head way back, or to focus on the bend in the lower back, but these don't have a great effect on the crucial knot at the heart. Get in touch with the feel of the skin streching across your chest; you'll want to have this item on your checklist during the Longbow especially.

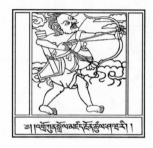

When you're in the Arrow, be aware first of the stretch in the balls of your feet, your instep, and the calves. This is very refreshing after a day on your feet. The muscles of the back of the foot and lower leg are also connected in a long chain all the way to our upper back and shoulders, and so you might feel afterward as if you've just had a good back rub.

Opening your mouth during this part of the exercise is the Lion Pose. Open wider and wider until you feel two parallel lines of stretching skin going up and down on either side of your nose and mouth. Keep this stretch going all through the five breaths.

Those two side channels that run up alongside the central channel at the spine continue up the back of our neck to the top of the head, and then come down the forehead. At the spot between our eyebrows, they twist around the central channel and form a small but nasty knot. When you're trying to concentrate, or get upset about something, and then squish up this same spot in the middle of your lower forehead, it's actually that little knot, tightening up even worse. That's also why headaches seem so often to start at our forehead.

When we stretch the sides of our mouth in the Lion Pose, it actually tugs at the ends of the two side channels running down next to our nostrils. This loosens the knot at the forehead and relieves tension accumulated there throughout the day.

There's something else that's very important to know about these two loose ends of the side channels. One powerful way to stretch them out and loosen up the forehead knot is simply a big honest smile. No kidding; that's one of the reasons why smiling feels so good in the first place.

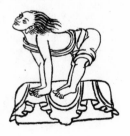

Rounding your back at the end of the Arrow balances out all the backward bending. Scrunch up your shoulders, and feel the skin stretching in a strip across

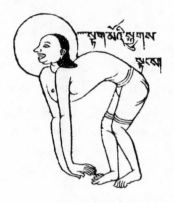

your upper back. You might hear slight crackling sounds and then tension being released from your neck and shoulders in a pleasant stream. Little sounds like this during the exercises are a good sign: Tiny jets of inner wind are being released while a minor knot slips open for an instant. As your yoga practice progresses, you'll hear fewer and fewer of these little cracks, because the inner channels begin to open and stay open.

This brings us to an important part of yoga that isn't much talked about. The exercises at level one—the level of our physical body—function to facilitate the flow of inner wind through the various subtle channels. This is the whole point of yoga poses as they were originally intended.

Think of your inner channels like little garden hoses with knots in them. Suppose there's no water coming out of a hose, because there's a knot. And then maybe you don't notice the knot, and you go and turn the faucet wide open. You could burst the hose.

The same sort of thing can happen when you do some vigorous yoga, which sends more and more inner wind racing through the channels. If you haven't made an equal effort to loosen up the knots in the channels, you can get some unexpected results. These can range anywhere from a pulled muscle to feelings of irritability or competitiveness as you do more and more yoga.

Every student of yoga needs to work on avoiding this

problem—it can undo all the efforts we make in our yoga classes. The best way to work on the knots is simply to be very serious in the practice of Giving and Taking as you go through a session. Concentrate on the exhale of your breath—especially as you explode the air out with the sound of "ha" at the end of the Arrow. Send out the gift of joyful effort.

You know that wonderful feeling you get when you're excited about something you're working on—the creative juices are flowing, and there's a kind of excitement in the air. Your mind sinks into the task, and sleep or food might be forgotten for many hours at a time.

What we give upon the breath of the rose and the light of the diamond in this exercise is exactly that same kind of joyful excitement, in doing the most exciting thing in life: helping other people. Imagine that the person you're sending your gift to is suddenly inspired to be a Mother Teresa, in little things, to everyone around them all the time. Helping others a bit here and a bit there, all through the day, in your home or office: handing out kindnesses like Christmas gifts, all year long. Your knots won't be able to resist the joy you plant. The winds that your yoga stirs up will flow so free.

When we see a cow,
We are really
looking at
The opposite
of everything
That is not
the cow.

—Master Dharma Kirti
(7th Century)

EXERCISE •8•

Stillness

with

the sky

Much of the ultimate goal of the yoga exercises
is not only to make the inner winds flow more freely, but also
to make specific currents of inner wind flow in a different
direction. This has a profound effect on the very way we think,
opening up a whole new vision of everything around us. We'll
talk much more of that in the last two exercises; the process

begins here on the physical level with bringing our feet up over our heads, to the sky.

The standard Indian pose here is called "the Pose for All the Body" (*Sarvanga Asana*), because it is targeted at the entire body at once—especially the central core running up and down our very being. The bones of the neck are also loosened and opened, relieving the tie-up in the channels there.

The accompanying Tibetan pose is called "the Rag Doll" (*Kekap Chak*), a countermotion to even out the stretch of the neck before. It comes from one of the older lineages of Tibet. The point here is that we let go of all the tenseness in our neck and heart, allowing the shoulders, neck, and upper back to flop like a rag doll.

How to Do the Exercise

- Time: 3 minutes.
- Come again to a comfortable seated position.
- Inhale and say, "I send you stillness."
- Sit quietly for five cycles of exhale/inhale, sending the light and breath.
- *Out-breath:* Begin the All-Body Pose by exhaling and lying down on your back, with your legs outstretched.
- *In-breath:* Take your legs over your head, toward the floor behind you, keeping your legs together. Interlock your fingers and pull your shoulder blades toward each other. Then bend your elbows and place your palms side by side against your upper back, with your fingers pointing up toward the sky. Try to bring your elbows as close together as you can, and exhale.

- *In-breath:* Lean your back against your hands and raise your legs up until they are as perpendicular to the floor as possible. Make sure that your feet are directly over your hips and that most of your body's weight is resting on your shoulders, not on your neck. Fix your gaze just past your nose.

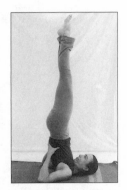

Pose for All the Body

- Remain here for fifteen cycles of exhale/inhale. Later, when you become accustomed to the pose, you can increase the number of cycles to 25.

- *Out-breath:* Lower your legs slowly down toward the floor behind you. You can either press your toes into the floor with the legs straight, or bend your knees beside your ears. Remain here for five cycles of exhale/inhale.

- *Out-breath:* Bend your knees and slowly roll down to a lying position on the mat. Inhale.

- Take five slow breaths, and then come to a standing position on your mat.

- Begin the Rag Doll: Stand with your feet together, and interlock your fingers behind your back with straight arms. Exhale fully.

- *In-breath:* Bend backward from the heart, pulling your shoulder blades together and keeping your lower back straight. Let your head fall back, gazing upward. Pull your arms down toward the floor for a deeper stretch.

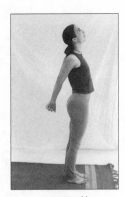

Rag Doll

- Remain here for five cycles of exhale/inhale.
- Release the pose, and come again to a sitting position on your mat.

How the Exercise Works on You

On a physical level, our heart works constantly to pump blood through miles of blood veins. The very beating of the heart is due to the flow of inner winds; the heart's shape reflects the configuration of ineffable channels in the same place. Our head is above our heart nearly the entire day, and the heart works extra hard to send blood straight up. Whenever we lie down, putting the head and heart on the same level, the heart takes a welcome break from fighting gravity. When we put the head *below* the heart, our brain gets a richer supply of food than ever.

Several of the exercises of Heart Yoga involve placing the head below the heart. At first this will feel unfamiliar and even a little uncomfortable. But after a few weeks you'll notice something happening. If you're one of those people who is plagued by a stuffed-up or runny nose much of the day, or if you have trouble with your sinuses—even hay fever or asthma— you'll soon find these exercises are a cheap, lasting alternative to

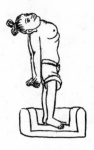 all those pills and sprays. Much of our congestion is simply due to gravity causing mucus to settle into pockets at the bottom of the sinuses. When the head comes down in a pose, this collected liquid is released, and by the end of the session we're breathing freely without even noticing it.

When the All-Body Pose is done correctly, you feel a sense of silence and balance—sometimes it feels almost as if you were flying. Doing the pose correctly of course takes some practice, and because it involves opening up the neck you should only begin it under the guidance of a qualified yoga instructor. But if you simply plug away at the exercise steadily for a few weeks, your neck will feel better than it has for many years.

It's also important that, after bending the neck forward, you balance this effort by bending it back; again, this prevents soreness after your yoga session. That's why, in Heart Yoga, we move on to the Rag Doll. Be sure to take a few breaths before standing up; the heart needs to readjust to pumping blood up to the head, and you might feel dizzy if you don't give it some time.

The very act of balancing can make us more aware of the invisible central channel—make it an item on your checklist at this point to try to "feel" it, a sense of centeredness. Continue to breathe as always with an emphasis on long, steady exhales made with that sound of a contented sigh. Here and during all the moving exercises the eyes remain open, gazing at the recommended spot, focused on a single point.

Focus is in fact what we are offering to that special person as we breathe out during this exercise. One form of focus is simply the extraordinary concentration that we see in a professional baseball player's eyes as he watches a fastball approach the plate. Or the look that

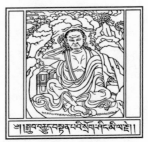

Tibet's greatest meditator, Milarepa (1040–1123)

a competent businesswoman gets during a tough negotiation on her cell phone.

At a deeper level, focus changes to meditation—a kind of single-pointed silence. It's not really much different from the absorbed feeling you get as you lose yourself in a good book or even a very engrossing movie. All these forms of concentration have one thing in common: We focus on *one* thing by eliminating all the other things around us. As the ancient masters said, when we see a single thing we are actually looking at the opposite of everything in the whole world that is *not* this thing. But now what's that got to do with yoga?

On a very basic level, it means that we can concentrate on an exercise better if there are *fewer* other objects in the room to cancel out. And all that means is that the place where you do your yoga should be clean and tidy—stow away or throw away everything in the room that you don't absolutely need, anything that could catch your eye and mind and pull them away from your single point of focus.

But this tidiness needs to happen on a wider scale if you ever hope to find the kind of concentration that we're sending to others here. That's because our minds are like a computer—they only have a certain capacity to store things, and no more. If I ask you how many pairs of shoes you have, or how many knickknacks scattered around your house, your mind immediately begins calling up pictures of each one of them. This demonstrates how cluttered our minds really are: Some old pair of tennis shoes that we never wear is taking up precious space in our minds. And if that seat is occupied when our next great idea needs a place to sit down, we might lose it altogether.

The same thing applies to our relationships, and the books

we read, and the news we choose to listen to. The capacity of the mind is not infinite. Relating to a hundred objects on a very shallow level prevents you from going deeply into one or two. And something happens to the inner winds when we do go deep: The flow begins to quiet down and clean up.

This has an immediate effect up on the first level, because a stretch of uninterrupted inner silence is infinitely more nutritious for the body than the old three square meals. Certain masters of yoga in ancient India and Tibet went beyond all need of food or even breathing; they lived on stillness alone.

We don't have to go that far, but you get the point. We need silent focus as much as we need food, if we want yoga to work for us and make us strong and trim. And so we give the stillness away to someone else, which is the best way to keep it: The seeds are planted.

EXERCISE •9•

The Death of Unknowing

Verses about yoga written more than six hundred years ago advise us to lie down quietly after a yoga session, to "calm the body and refresh the mind." The classic resting position is known as the Dead Man's Pose (*Shava Asana*), because physically the goal is to lie as still as a corpse.

Mentally we are still giving, still working from the inside. At the end of the exercise we do a brief pose from the tradition of the Dalai Lamas known as Shake & Stretch (*Trukdreng*), followed by a quiet moment of taking pleasure in the goodness of what we've tried to do with our yoga session.

How to Do the Exercise

- Time: 4 minutes.
- Begin the Dead Man's Pose: Lie down on your mat and let your arms and legs fall comfortably out to the sides. Keep the palms of your hands facing up, and the fingers relaxed. Lengthen your neck and pull your head away from the rest of the body, then let it relax,

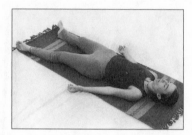

Dead Man's Pose

  closing your eyes. You can cover yourself with a blanket if you like.
- Breathe slowly out and in, and feel the weight of your body sink into the floor. Find any tension that you have in your body and let it go—picture it dissolving into the floor. Concentrate on this for about two minutes.
- Then, lying relaxed and quiet, take a breath in and say, "I send you wisdom."
- Remain still like this for two more minutes, sending the breath and light.
- Next do the Shake & Stretch. Slowly start to move your

hands and feet, stretching
them and shaking them out.
Turn your head from side to
side on the floor.

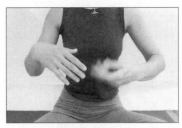

Shake & Stretch,
shaking out hands

- Take hold of each of the
  fingers of the right
  hand with the left, and
  one by one pull gently
  at the joints. Then switch
  and do the fingers of the
  other hand.

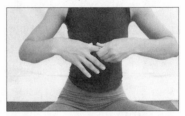

Shake & Stretch,
pulling joints

- Knead each palm and finger
  with the thumb of the
  opposite hand.

- Wring out your hands as if
  you were washing them.

- Now slowly turn onto your side, and push
  yourself up with your hands to a seated
  position.

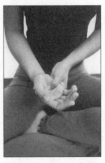

Shake & Stretch,
kneading hands

- Sit quietly for a moment. Remember the
  six gifts you have given, from the diamond
  and the rose at your heart. Be happy that
  you have tried to make someone else
  happy.

- Gaze one last time at the bridge of soft-
  blue light between your diamond and theirs. For a moment,
  just a moment, imagine that there are countless bridges of
  light like this between your heart and the hearts of every
  single living being, on every single planet in the entire
  universe.

How the Exercise Works on You

In this final exercise on the mat, we strive simply to relax every single part of our body. It's a well-earned rest, but you may discover that you begin to tense up at the usual places, just by habit. Put it on your mental checklist to stay vigilant, looking for spots that still need to relax.

There should be a change here at the second level, in your breathing. Relax the part of the throat that helped you make the sighing noise up to now, but still let the air sweep over the same spot in your throat, both on the out-breath and the in-breath. This helps the inner winds flow better in all three major channels, at the back of the neck. Try now to make long and very silent breaths.

Take some time to think about all five levels; you can even picture yourself dropping down through each of them, deep into your body. Be aware of the physical body relaxing and the quieting of the breath. Follow the quiet breath down to the inner winds; see if you can actually feel them. Don't look for something that feels like the air from a fan going through a soda straw. The inner winds as they sing now through the inner channels are much more likely to feel like the simple contentment you experience as you sit quietly on the side of a forest mountain, or at the edge of the sea at night.

Come down now to your thoughts, riding on these gentle new

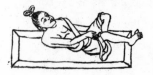 winds. Think about the final gift: the gift of wisdom, the gift of knowing important things, the deeper things of life.

Of course, wisdom comes in as many flavors as ice cream does. What we're talking about here is a very specific kind of wisdom.

Wherever the Dalai Lama goes, whatever he says, he repeats one thing over and over. Despite all the differences between the people on this Earth, we are all the same in one way. We all want things to go well for us,

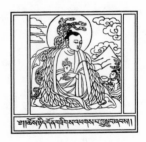

Naga Arjuna
(3rd century),
Master of Wisdom

and nobody wants any of the problems or trouble of life. But problems and trouble do come to us; we are never free of them for very long. Wisdom is understanding where these problems really come from, and how to stop them.

All through our session of Tibetan Heart Yoga so far, we've been trying to plant new good seeds in our minds, by thinking kind thoughts, even as we work on our body. If you do your yoga this way—patiently, happily, day after day—then your mental supply of good seeds grows and grows.

Remember that, according to the greatest wisdom of the masters of ancient India and Tibet, these seeds ripen in our minds and color how we see both everything around us and everything about us. If we have been kind and considerate toward others, then these seeds come back to us later. They color how we see our very world; for example, you may find the weather, whatever it is, more and more enjoyable. They color how we see other people: You'll discover that fewer and fewer people annoy you through the day. They color even how we see ourselves: Your yoga begins to *work* on you—you feel stronger, younger, and simply a lot happier than ever before.

Ballerinas,

When you stand

at a bus stop

Practice, quietly,

That turn of

the foot.

—George Balanchine
(1904–1983), greatest
ballet master of the
20th Century

EXERCISE • 10 •

All-Day

Yoga

So half an hour of Heart Yoga every day plants a ton of
wonderful world-seeds in our mind. But it's not hard to see
that—if we just let the other twenty-three and a half hours of
the day go the same old way—it's not very likely that we'll be
able to avoid the same old mix of good and bad seeds as we
interact with others. And then our days will continue to be an

unpredictable mix of ups and downs; we'll never get rid of all the problems that spoil our life.

This is where the idea of All-Day Yoga comes in. In Tibetan it's called *Chulam Neljor*. Some of the greatest descriptions of it are found in the writings of a master called Quicksilver Dharma Bhadra (1772–1851) and in works by Dechen Nyingpo (1878–1941), the teacher of the teacher of His Holiness the current Dalai Lama.

The way to do All-Day Yoga is simply to slip back to one of the five levels at odd moments throughout the day—whenever you think of it—whether you're at home, or at work, or somewhere in between. You do a little touch of yoga and then go on with your day. Let's see how this works at each of the five levels.

Physically the most important form of All-Day Yoga is simply sitting up straight, all day long, no matter what you're doing. Don't think this is as trivial as it sounds. In ancient Tibet, sitting straight all day was considered one of the most important yoga practices of all. It's imperative, if we want to be healthy and strong, that the central channel remain as straight and free of kinks as possible all day long. If the spine slumps, the central channel goes with it.

It's also important to keep your shoulders from scrunching in throughout the day. This scrunching is a natural reaction to the pressures of life, and at some point our shoulders begin to stick in this position. That constricts the knot behind the heart, blocking off our inner winds and inhibiting our full capacity to truly love all the people around us.

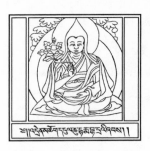

Master Dharma Bhadra

As you delve deeper into yoga, you'll begin to experience something called the "inner locks." These are methods of purposely directing the inner winds and breaking through the knots in the channels. You can start working on one of them now, throughout the day. And again it's simply remembering to tuck your tummy in, as you walk or stand or sit.

With time, you'll feel special, subtle muscles farther down your abdomen that you tense lightly, creating a spot of inner silence that has a very beautiful influence on the inner winds. For now, just suck in your stomach very lightly and gently, whenever you think of it during the day. Doing this doesn't hurt your waistline either; and incidentally, it's a lot easier to do if your back is straight and your shoulders are pulled slightly back, opening your chest and heart to the world.

Don't forget to work on the two side channels too, by pulling up the corners of your mouth: Smile, as much as you can, every minute of the day.

On the next level down, the breath, come back constantly during your working day to simply *exhaling* fully and slowly. Doing this will take care of everything else and prevent that jerky, nearly panting breath that often comes to us when we're slightly under pressure at the office or at home. This helps us avoid any disturbances of the inner winds at the next level down—disturbances that cause most work-related disease: ulcers, heart problems, and disorders related to long periods at a computer.

Remember though that the very best way to get to these inner winds is from the fourth level down: the thoughts. If you keep nothing else from this little book, let it be the extraordinary skill of doing Giving and Taking all day long. As

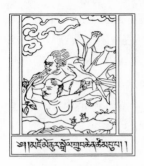

ༀ །མི་ཆོས་ཆུ་རུ་སྙོལ་བྱུང་བ་ཆེན་ཚོ་མ་ལུ་པ །

One day a monk
stopped to help an
old woman with
leprosy. She turned
into an angel and
took him to heaven.

you travel to work and are stuck in a traffic jam, look ahead—at the back of the head in the car that just cut in front of you. Put your loving eyes on that tired businessman slumped across from you in the subway. Glance at the person in your office who's obviously stressed out today. Look at your husband, or your wife, or your child—anyone you take for granted—having a difficult evening at home.

And then just quietly, silently, anonymously, breathe. Just sit there and breathe. Breathe the air in softly, take the trouble from their heart, take it into your diamond and destroy every bit of it. Breathe out, and give them whatever you think they might want or need. A day off? A raise? A pet? A friend, to stop the loneliness? Patience? Health? Wisdom? Feel the fragrance from the rose brush against them; touch their diamond with a ray of light from your own. And then in the next instant, as the traffic light changes or the subway empties out, just go on your way. This is true yoga; the seeds are truly planted.

Until the day
That the
sky itself,
With all the
sun and stars,

Falls down
to earth
May I remain
To help every
living being.

—Traditional Tibetan
prayer often quoted by
His Holiness the Dalai Lama

Changing Spears to Flowers

You should know, before we finish this book, *why* the ancient sages in the tradition of the Dalai Lamas did yoga in the first place. Each one of us, they would say, has come to this world for a purpose. Everything that we do in this life should help us fulfill the real purpose that was meant for us.

We can use yoga to make us healthy and strong—trim and

attractive—and that's a good thing. It's no fun to feel run down, or to get old, and there's nothing wrong with wanting to look your best. But once you've achieved all this with yoga—and you can, with half an hour of steady work every day—then you'll feel like you want to go on. We were meant for more.

It's one thing to imagine that we could help others; and as you get better at Giving and Taking, you must begin to do it not only for friends and family, but also for strangers and even for people you may not like so much. And certainly this wonderful breathing practice can refresh our own hearts like nothing else, planting powerful seeds to bring us health and calmness. But still—and you know it deep down in your own heart—we want more. We were meant for more.

We want it to come true. We want to really be able to help every single person there is. Not just pretending—we want the real thing. But we have only two hands; we're stuck in one little body of flesh and bone, in one little part of a big, mixed-up world. How could we ever really help everyone else? For this is our destiny, this is what each one of us was meant to do; we sense it, and we cannot really ever be satisfied until we reach it.

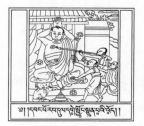

Changing spears
to flowers

Now that you've read about how Tibetan Heart Yoga works, and now that you've tried a little of it, you'll be able to guess for yourself how the dream can come true. Over two thousand years ago, a young prince sat beneath a tree in India, on the edge of a great change. Thousands of evil spirits rushed forward to stop the change. They threw spears at him; they shot arrows to kill him. But halfway through the air, before they ever touched him, the spears and arrows changed to beautiful flowers, a shower of fragrant blooms. They changed.

We will change too. If we continue, with mule-like patience, to do the yoga of Giving and Taking, day after quiet day, and all day long, then slowly the new seeds will take over from the old ones. You know how the seeds can ripen and color what we see—you know they can make you see the boss walk in smiling instead of yelling. You know they will make you see your body differently, as you do your yoga and become more strong and healthy. But why stop there?

If a single thing in the world can change—if world-seeds can make a single joint in a sore back stop hurting—then *anything* can change. If you can walk one step, you can walk ten; it's just more of the same. Yoga in ancient times wasn't designed to stop at making us healthy, just so we could take longer to die. It was meant to change *everything*. It was meant to take each one of us on to what we are really meant be.

It will come to you, and you will know it when it comes. At all five levels, we change—we change *completely*. The seeds change our thoughts, the thoughts change the winds. The winds change the channels, and the channels

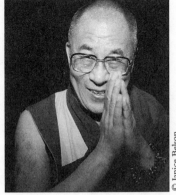

© Janice Belson

change the body. You cannot go to every world, and to every hurting person in every world, with a body like the one we have now. As the last change comes, you will become like the light of the diamond itself. Then go, and give them all they need.

Advice for Your Daily Session, and Finding Out More

Before starting any yoga program, you should always get a checkup from your doctor or other health provider. Describe the kind of activities you'll be doing, especially if you have any existing medical conditions. The best guide, of course, is common sense. As with so many things, you are much more likely to succeed with Tibetan Heart Yoga if you just take it slow but steady—a steady flow of practice, every day.

It is good to take one day off a week as a break, almost to savor the practice. Take the *same* day off each week, and also try to start your practice at exactly the same time every day. Your body and mind will then begin to get into a very regular rhythm. In time, you'll notice that your system even adjusts the timing of your bowel movements so that your bowels are cleared before your daily session. You'll find that all such cycles—digestion, elimination, and even menstruation—become very regular and easy.

Your yoga sessions will be much more productive if your stomach is empty—try not to eat anything for at least three hours before practice, and after a session wait for half an hour before eating. Juice or water is fine not long before or after; for people who tend toward low blood sugar, juice can prevent any dizziness. Coffee or tea with caffeine before a session is simply a bad idea, because of the effect on your heart and breathing.

The big challenge, as always, will be to keep your practice going steadily. You can't expect great results if you work very hard for a few days a week and then do nothing on the other days. Better a steady, modest effort every day.

One way to keep on track is to do your sessions at home with a friend or family member: your spouse, child, or parent. It's very good if you can get to the local yoga school too, once or twice a week. Again, many of the physical exercises of Heart Yoga are being done at almost every yoga school around the country. Take the time to make sure the teacher is really qualified, and then listen carefully to their instructions and incorporate these right away into your daily routine.

Don't try to rush or shorten your session—give it a good, full half hour a day. If you find yourself short of time, then sit down purposely and make a clear decision about some other activity that you do on a regular basis, and that you might cut short or eliminate, to make room for the yoga.

Most people find it easier to do Heart Yoga in the morning, when they're fresh, but everybody's body clock is different. Experiment and see what's best for you. Yoga in general is difficult to do when you haven't had enough sleep—don't start too late in the evening, and most important make sure that you get whatever amount of sleep you really need. You may be able to "cheat" at work if you haven't gotten enough sleep, by drinking extra cups of coffee. But caffeine doesn't fool the inner channels.

Stay warm during your practice sessions, and afterward too. Avoid cold floors; we recommend a standard "sticky" foam mat with a traditional cotton mat placed over it—this is warmer and cleaner, and prevents the plastic from coming into direct contact with your skin.

For this reason too it's good during your practice to wear clothes that are either entirely or mostly made of natural fibers like cotton or wool. They should not be so tight that they pinch in when you fold over or turn. Nor should they be so loose that they obstruct your face or breathing when you bend down, or that you find yourself catching on them as you move.

Don't overpush to make a stretch, or lose form to try to look good. Stay in the posture and alignment of your body that you know is correct, and then simply stretch as far as you can comfortably. Find and remain quietly in that steady gentle tension of a muscle as you stretch it.

Be patient; progress in the physical exercises is made in tiny increments of a fraction of an inch, over a long period of regular daily practice. It's much more important to maintain your thoughts of Giving and Taking on the inside and calm steady breathing—especially on the out-breaths. If you find yourself puffing or feeling anxious or have difficulty getting enough air, back off a bit on the pose, until your breathing is smooth and you feel calm.

You'll feel sore after your sessions for the first few weeks. Expect this and enjoy it. The old creaky channels are opening up. If something hurts, though, stop immediately and talk to a qualified yoga teacher—almost always it's because you're not doing something the right way, and this can be fixed in a matter of minutes.

Most important, have fun during your sessions. Don't let them become a chore. If you feel this happening, you need to crank up your Giving and Taking, especially during the day— helping others anonymously with your breath.

Move with grace and dignity, like a ballet dancer. You're going to feel awkward for the first few weeks, but after that you'll be glad the whole rest of your life for the wonderful energy you get from the practice. Don't worry about what other people think about your new project; they'll poke fun at you and then they'll be doing Heart Yoga themselves shortly, after they see what it does for you.

And don't make the mistake of comparing yourself to other people who practice. Go at your own steady pace; each body is different, and some take time to "turn on" to the yoga. Many, many yoga students who started late and awkward, but who were patient and steady in their practice, have succeeded where those with "natural" bodies and abilities flashed and faded away. Tibetan Heart Yoga also knows no age; you can and should start no matter how old or young you are.

A lot of people who try Heart Yoga begin to get great results and want to know if they can delve deeper into it. The half-hour practice you find here is the core of all practices, and you can find something deeper in it every day for a whole lifetime.

The tradition does indeed have many further levels, each one tailored to the special needs and abilities of each different type of person. It's also very important to have a real, live person to guide you through the ins and outs of a typical Heart Yoga session, to check your progress, and to suggest ways you can get even more out of your efforts. Many helpful details can be communicated only by what the Tibetan masters call *shel-shey*: from mouth to ear, and not from the dry pages of a book.

And so it can be very good for the growth of your practice if you find an instructor who is qualified to teach Tibetan Heart Yoga in the traditional way. If you would like to find out about a teacher or a Tibetan Heart Yoga Center or visiting seminar in your area—or even if you just have a question to ask or want to talk—please contact us at www.HeartYoga.org. It would be our pleasure to get to know you and pass the tradition on to you— and then too you can help pass it on to others.

Acknowledgments

We would like to thank His Holiness the Dalai Lama for being in our world, as an example for us to follow.

We would like to thank all the Tibetan lamas who have tirelessly guided us for many years. First among these is Khen Rinpoche Geshe Lobsang Tharchin, founder of the MSTC Tibetan Buddhist centers and former abbot of Sera Mey

Tibetan Monastery. He has devoted thousands upon thousands of hours in passing on these traditions freely, to both Tibetans and westerners around the world.

Geshe Lobsang Thardo and Geshe Thupten Rinchen of Sera Mey imparted countless lessons to us. Geshe Trinley Topgye, former abbot of the Gyumey Tibetan Tantric College and also a teacher at Sera Mey, took us carefully through many subjects. Dozens of other master monks from Sera Mey have helped us as well.

Lama Zopa Rinpoche, director of the FPMT global network of Tibetan Buddhist centers, has been a lifetime inspiration to all of us and has helped bring this wisdom to the entire world.

We are deeply indebted to many masters of the modern yoga tradition, flowing as it does from ancient India. Masters David Life and Sharon Gannon, founders of the Jivamukti method, have showered us with their wisdom and skill in every aspect of yoga. Lady Ruth Lauer, also from Jivamukti, showed us yoga with devotion and love for others. We are also deeply indebted to the fine teachers Carolyn Christie (Iyengar tradition), Pilar Settlemeir (Ashtanga), Lisa Schrempp (Ashtanga), and David Swenson (Ashtanga). Each of these western masters has truly carried on the work of their own Indian teachers—among them Shri Swami Shivananda, Shri K. Pattabhi Jois, and Shri B.K.S. Iyengar—to whom we also offer endless gratitude.

None of this work would have been possible without the many classes in Sanskrit language granted to us freely over the years by Professor Samuel D. Atkins, chairman emeritus of the Department of Classics of Princeton University.

John Brady, director of the Asian Classics Input Project, supplied many valuable materials for the book, often through the indefatigable efforts of the Project's manager of South Asian Operations, Geshe Ngawang Rigdol. Other quite rare yoga manuscripts came as a result of the many years of work by the ACIP research team in Russia, including especially Ngawang Kheatsun and Jampa Namdol. Professor Lev Serafimovich Savitsky and Dr. Vladimir Uspensky, of the Oriental Library of the St. Petersburg branch of the Russian Academy of Sciences, have helped guide this team selflessly over many years' time.

Several experts in modern physiology and movement theory have helped us clarify the connection between the physical body and the inner body presented in the Tibetan traditions. These include Professor Ze'eva Cohen, chairman of the Department of Dance, Princeton University; Laura Donnelly of the University of Arizona's Department of Dance; and Allison Cohen, of the Dingman school of the Balanchine method of ballet.

It would be impossible to list here all the other individuals who have helped make this presentation of Heart Yoga a reality; we thank all of you once again, including trisangma for modelling the exercise photos so beautifully; Amber Moore for illustration work; Angela Bleackley, Brian Pearson, and Jenny Thomas for proofreading; David Fishman, Matthew Gerson, and Mira Shani for testing the poses; Andrea and Ted Lemon for logistical support; Janice Allen and Jim Davidson for great meals; and Ziggy for hugs and going outside.

Last but certainly not least, we would like to thank Mr. Trace Murphy, our editor at Doubleday, for his vision, his faith in the work of saving and recording these traditions, and his relentless demand that we pursue excellence in presenting them.

About the Authors

The Diamond Mountain teachers are a group of teachers from the United States, Ireland, Canada, and Australia who have extensively studied the ancient wisdom traditions of Tibet and India with the great masters. Geshe Michael Roach originated the text and completed the major part of the translation of the ancient scriptures used for reference in *The*

Tibetan Book of Yoga. This manuscript was then edited and prepared for publication by members of the Diamond Mountain team. All of the Diamond Mountain teachers listed here are certified to conduct seminars and talks about the methods described in this book. If you would like to arrange a presentation in your area, please contact www.HeartYoga.org.

Geshe Michael Roach is the first American to complete the twenty-year course in a traditional Tibetan monastery and earn the title of "Geshe," or Master of Buddhism. He is the founder of the Asian Classics Input Project, which is probably the world's largest database of ancient Asian manuscripts, and the author of several internationally selling popular books on Eastern spirituality. He is a translator of Sanskrit and Tibetan and recently completed a three-year deep meditation retreat in the Arizona desert.

Kimberley Anderson-Veenhof is an international business consultant and personal coach. She travels extensively, conducting training workshops based on Enlightened Business Institute principles (www.enlightenedbusiness.com). She is a long-term yoga student and teaches Authentic Dance.

Giselle Ansselin is a cofounder of Australia's Diamond Cutter Buddhist Centre, and a popular teacher of the Asian Classics Institute course series. She is a social worker and naturopath in the area of holistic health.

Mercedes Bahleda is a graduate of the Experimental Theater Wing at New York University. As a professional dancer, actor, and singer, she has toured widely in Europe and the United States. She has done extensive deep retreat work and has been a student of yoga for six years.

John Brady is director of the Asian Classics Input Project, an international project to save the endangered sacred literature of Tibet. He is also a senior teacher at the Asian Classics Institute of New York, and a former sales director at the Lillian Vernon Company of New York.

Deborah Bye is a barrister from Melbourne, Australia, and discovered Tibetan Buddhism in her twenties, while traveling in India. Her background includes hatha yoga, vipassana meditation, and Kashmir Shaivism, as well as the classic Buddhist scriptures. She is the coordinator of a project to teach Buddhist philosophy, meditation, and yoga in prisons in the United States.

Nancy Carin is a mother of three and founder of the Business Outreach Center of New York. She is a longtime instructor of tai chi and also a popular teacher at the Asian Classics Institute in Manhattan.

James Connor is a CEO with a spiritual approach to business and life. His brand strategy agency, the James Group, is run entirely on the Buddhist principles of causation and serving others. He is an active teacher in New York City as director of Godstow Meditation Retreat Center, and as director of the Pate Institute for Peace.

Ian Davies is a cofounder of Australia's Diamond Cutter Centre, where he teaches the courses of the Asian Classics Institute. He is a longtime practitioner of shiatsu therapy and yoga.

Anthony Deague is a graduate of the University of Melbourne and works for a large property corporation. He has studied at the Asian Classics Institute and with many Tibetan masters in Australia, and currently coordinates the study program at a Tibetan Buddhist center in Melbourne. Formerly a professional athlete, Anthony conducts yoga classes for sporting clubs and school groups.

Gail Deutsch coordinates the public teachings at Diamond Mountain. She discovered Tibetan Buddhism in India during her twenties, and then traveled to Tibet. She has studied closely with major Tibetan lamas, including Lama Zopa Rinpoche, and has helped found a number of dharma centers.

Michael O'Reilly Dunn is an information technology specialist, currently serving as senior manager and director at Riskforce, based in Ireland and the United States. He holds degrees in IT from the School of Visual Arts, New York, and from NYU's Tisch School of the Arts. He is a student of both Tibetan Buddhism and Ashtanga yoga.

Alistair Holmes was born in the United Kingdom; he completed his undergraduate degree in political philosophy from the University of Queensland, Australia, and then worked in the legal profession. He is a director of a large private investment company, and has studied at both Diamond Mountain and Sera Mey Tibetan Monastery.

Venerable Konchok Kyizom is a nun in the Tibetan Buddhist tradition. She leads a successful psychology practice in her native Canada, as well as teaching ballet and yoga. She also heads classes in the Asian Classics Institute course series, and has studied at Sera Mey Tibetan Monastery.

Salim Lee is a teacher who has been sharing his knowledge and practice with many students in Australia, Asia, Europe, and the United States. He is an architect, builder, and property developer specializing in aged care, as well as a college professor and father of three children.

Anne Lindsey (Venerable Lobsang Chukyi) is an ordained Buddhist nun and teacher with studies at a major Tibetan monastery and a doctoral-level education in clinical psychology at the City College of New York. She has worked as a supervising psychologist for school-based counseling programs in New York City.

Andrea McCullough is a specialist in spiritual dance forms, with performances in the United States and Europe. She integrates her studies and yoga practice with raising young children and teaching them a spiritual path.

Winston McCullough has studied at a major Tibetan Buddhist monastery, and is director of Diamond Mountain, a thousand-acre study and meditation center in Arizona. He has served as a business consultant for eighteen years, has been a professor of business management at Columbia University, and is a popular teacher in the United States, Asia, and Europe.

Christie McNally has studied yoga with some of the world's most renowned masters, and has trained in several major Tibetan monasteries. She is a Tibetan and Sanskrit translator and textual expert with the Asian Classics Input Project. She recently completed a three-year deep retreat in the Arizona desert.

Ani Pelma (Venerable Debra Ballier) is founder of the Three Jewels, a popular Manhattan bookstore and outreach center. She translates Tibetan texts, has also studied at Sera Mey, and is a prizewinning poet. Having finished a three-year deep retreat, she currently serves as a retreat master at Diamond Mountain.

Elizabeth Prather is the founder of a successful yoga tour company. Prior to that she worked in the management of several HMO corporations. She is a longtime student of Tibetan Buddhism, having studied at Tibetan monasteries in both India and Nepal.

Brian Smith is a professor at the University of California, Riverside. He specializes in religious studies and the Sanskrit language, and has published a number of books and major translations from Sanskrit with both the Oxford University Press and Penguin Books. He has studied extensively in India, and at Sera Mey Tibetan Monastery. He is also a popular teacher of the ACI courses in the Los Angeles area.

John Stilwell is director of the Asian Classics Institute of New York, where thousands of people have trained, and was the founding director of Godstow Retreat Center. He worked as a corporate executive and on Wall Street for nineteen years. He has taught in the United States and Europe for almost twenty years.

David K. Stumpf has a Ph.D. in plant biochemistry, and is a military historian. He has completed all eighteen courses offered by the Asian Classics Institute, and now teaches his own students in both the United States and South Africa. He is a member of the Board of Trustees of Diamond Mountain.

Susan Stumpf, David's wife, has trained as a physician assistant specializing in acupuncture and energetic/spiritual healing, including studies in Hong Kong. She has also completed the Asian Classics Institute course series, and now teaches ACI classes in the United States.

Kevin Thornton is the father of four children and has led an extended career in secondary-school education in his native Ireland. He is a longtime student of spirituality and a founding member of the Diamond Bay Buddhist Group of Galway, where he currently teaches the Asian Classics Institute courses.

Miriam Thornton, who is married to Kevin, is a lifetime follower of the spiritual path. She is a physiotherapist who has practiced yoga for many years, and now leads classes in Galway. She is also a founding member of the Diamond Bay Buddhist group.

Venerable Elly van der Pas is an ordained Buddhist nun and teacher with a master's degree in East-West Studies and several years of additional study and practice in Asian monasteries and ashrams. She is a former editor of *Mandala* magazine, and former development specialist with the Tibet Fund of His Holiness the Dalai Lama in New York.

Douglas Veenhof is an award-winning journalist and mountaineer guide who has guided extensively through Asia. He is a long-term student of Tibetan Buddhism, and former director of a dharma center in the North Cascades.

Rebecca Vinacour is a graduate of New York University's Tisch School of the Arts. She has studied extensively both at the Asian Classics Institute of New York and at Sera Mey Tibetan Monastery. She is enrolled in the Tibetan program at Diamond Mountain and practices the martial arts.

Rani Sheilagh Dunn (yogarani) is a cofounder of the Prana Yoga Centre in Dublin, Ireland. She has trained extensively in the Jivamukti and Devereux methods, with additional study under Shri B.K.S. Iyengar, Shri K. Pattabhi Jois, and David Swenson.